TRANSFORMED
═ O N E ═
W I N T E R

M A R S H A G. S P R A D L I N

BROADMAN PRESS
Nashville, Tennessee

ISBN: 0-8054-5076-9
Dewey Decimal Classification: B
Subject Heading: SPRADLIN, MARSHA G.
Library of Congress Catalog Card Number: 88-39527

Printed in the United States of America

Unless otherwise indicated, all Scripture quotations are from the HOLY BIBLE *New International Version,* copyright © 1978, New York Bible Society. Used by permission. Those marked (KJV) are from the King James Version of the Bible. Those marked (NASB) are from the *New American Standard Bible.* Copyright © The Lockman Foundation, 1960, 1962, 1963, 1968, 1971, 1972, 1973, 1975, 1977. Used by permission.

Library of Congress Cataloging-in-Publication Data

Spradlin, Marsha G., 1954-
    Transformed one winter / Marsha G. Spradlin.
        p.   cm.
    ISBN 0-8054-5076-9
    1. Spradlin, Marsha G., 1954-   . 2. Christian life—1960-
    3. Depression, Mental—Patients—United States—Biography.
    4. Sarcoidosis—Patients—United States—Biography.   I. Title.
BX6495.S67A3   1989
248.8'6'0924—dc 19
[B]   88-39527

Transformed One Winter
is dedicated to
ALL WHO HAVE TAUGHT ME LOVE!

To Mother and Daddy and my immediate family
for teaching me the meaning of love;

To Barbara Curnutt
for teaching me the meaning of friendship;

To Sarah and Ramon
for teaching me the meaning of acceptance;

To my doctors
for teaching me the meaning of compassion;

To Jeff Saunders
for teaching me the meaning of forgiveness;

To my co-workers
for teaching me the meaning of support;

To Cliff Temple Baptist Church, Dallas, Texas,
for teaching me the meaning of ministry

To the Father for teaching me the meaning of LIFE!

Acknowledgments

Special thanks to Mary Ann Ward Appling, Betty Merrell, and many friends who read this manuscript, made editorial suggestions, and encouraged me to share my story.

This is a true story based on the writer's personal journal, notes to Father, and correspondence with family and friends. Some names, including those of the physicians, have been changed to ensure their anonymity.

*Another book by Marsha G. Spradlin: *Livingtouch: Your Personal Witness in an Impersonal World* . . .

A Word at the Beginning

I remember the first time I saw Marsha. I had two overwhelming impressions: she is an attractive model of the contemporary women's leader, and she has it together. She knows where she wants to go and has a pretty good idea about how she's going to get there.

These were important impressions for me, for I carefully guard the positive image of our missions organization for women. The world needs to see the women of God as they are—competent, joyful, attractive, enthusiastic, confident.

My next impressions of Marsha confirmed the first. I came to know her, somewhat casually, as I observed her work with children and their leaders. She handled the responsibility and the challenge of leadership in Texas with expertise and vision.

Then I observed her as her body and spirit went through the throes of desperate illness. I called the leaders of our organization to prayer at specific times of the day. We were helpless in knowing how we could respond to her needs. But Marsha was not desperate. She was quietly and steadily engaged in a battle for life and hope, and her teacher, friend, guide, and physician was her Heavenly Father.

In the summer after her halting return to her work, she came to a huge meeting of high school girls. Seeing her behind stage,

I grabbed her frail body in a bear hug. With a start, I realized that although her physical body was frail, her spirit was gigantic. Any fleeting thought of pity left my mind. I have never since felt pity for Marsha: compassion, love, and support, always, but pity never.

For Marsha had found the reality of God, the great I AM. She had learned through hard lessons that He is sufficient for every need and circumstance. He was there for her, and that intimate, personal knowledge meant that she would never be weak, hopeless, desperate.

The day came when we invited Marsha to work in the national office of our organization. She arrived here with the same confidence I had seen in my first encounter with her. She brought a new zest for life and service to the organization for young adult women. Her calendar filled with engagements, for everyone wanted to experience her deep knowledge of missions and the Lord. Her committee and work-group assignments grew, for everyone wanted her creative ideas and team spirit. She wrote the manual that will guide this organization in the years ahead. She gave a positive, determined direction to the plans and activities for the age group.

Then the dread disease, systemic sarcoidosis, began to hammer again at her body. In response, Marsha began to write down her experiences of earlier days when her body was at total war with the sickness. She brought me a copy of the manuscript. I read it through without stopping, understanding for the first time what makes Marsha different. Yes, she wanted me to write the foreword, and she wanted my affirmation for the publishing. Those were minor decisions to make, but I also wanted her permission to share the book with my sister who, though not ill, was going through personal crisis. My sister's response was one of deep gratitude. Sharing with Marsha through her walk with the Lord, Eileen found her own path with the Lord.

Marsha Spradlin is an encourager. When she can hardly lift

her head, she remembers my situation and prays for me. Beyond that, she writes notes, encouraging, assuring, and pointing toward Scripture that suits the need I face.

Marsha is a positive Christian. Although some may think she is a mystic, she is a pragmatist. She knows that it works, this business of walking and talking with the Father.

Marsha is a communicator. Her message is clearly stated in terms and experiences that can be understood by people who are searching, too.

I am glad that she has written and is now being published. I am glad that others can enter her life and call her friend. Most of all, I am glad that the number of pray-ers will grow, as readers share with us the hymn of gratitude and praise: "It is of the Lord's mercies that we are not consumed, because his compassions fail not. They are new every morning: Great is thy faithfulness" (Lam. 3:22-23).

CAROLYN WEATHERFORD
Executive Director
Woman's Missionary Union, SBC

Contents

Prologue
A Time to Dance

Prologue

March 7, 1987—Orlando, Florida

Today is my birthday! And I am celebrating alone. A speaking engagement in Florida prevented me from being with family and friends. At one time, that would have been extremely disappointing. But, it really is OK. Certainly, I would prefer being with family today, but I realize that our love reaches beyond space and time. Our lives are more than bodies with souls. For that reason, my birthday celebration is different than it used to be. I celebrate not my thirty-three years of life but my three-year pilgrimage to find life, embrace all of it, and actually live it. Only three years ago today, my cradle swung over my own grave. I was dying.

My episode with dying was physical. The encounter with the mysterious, prolonged illness devastated my body and depleted my energy. Life was slowly sucked out, ounce by ounce, from my once active and physically fit body.

My episode with dying was emotional. How well I remember Jeff! I was in love. I thought I would never get over losing him. When I needed him the most, he was gone. His departure could not have come at a more serious time.

My episode with dying was professional. My doctor grounded me from traveling, and I thought this meant creating and living, also.

It is hard to imagine that was only three years ago. It's still harder to realize that three years and seven months ago, I felt totally in charge of my life. For the most part, life was going well. People described me as a woman who had everything. But by whose standards? I was a twenty-nine-year-old single, professional woman who owned her own home and car and enjoyed beautiful clothes, a fantastic job, a wonderful church, and caring Christian friends. My hopes and dreams would have made a good movie.

I accepted Jesus Christ as Lord and Savior as a sixteen-year-old high school sophomore. For many years I was an active church member and Sunday School teacher and had even spent summers as a counselor at one of my denomination's camps for girls. I felt my relationship with the Father was perfect! I was mistaken.

I remember the sudden change. With little warning, every hope and dream I had was all but snuffed out. My soul began to sink deep into the cavity of my own devastation. My only thought was: *How can I survive?* Not only was I dying, I had lost hope.

But the Father taught me the meaning of hope. We each can have it. I had it all along. I still cannot define it. At best, I can only describe it and experience it. I can't touch it, but I can certainly feel it. Hope is essential to life. Without it, I cease to thrive.

I am thankful for life and hope. At birth, the Father gave me these two. Life—it is fatal, and there are no exceptions. Hope—it will continue to convince me that I am the exception. Where is hope born? I remember my desperate feeling to escape quickly to that special place.

In my journey to find hope, I confronted questions about the quality of my life: Who was I created to be? What is the value of beauty? What is meaningful to me? What contributions have I made to the quality of life in others? These questions sank deep into my consciousness. In the storm of my winter, I promised myself and the Father that if I lived, I would never again identify who I am with where I am, what I do, or who I am with.

Life is more than that. It must encompass more than feelings, relationships, a job, or even physical beauty. In choosing to fight, the battle must not be to simply stay alive, but to direct my energy to choose to live *life!* Otherwise, there is no reason to fight. It took far more courage and energy to fight than simply give up and let my body do what would have been natural and a relief—to die.

What I have learned during the months and years that followed is worthy of divine celebration. It has been underscored with the conviction that holding on in the wind is harder than letting go. But holding on is the only way to hear His voice. He has spoken so much louder to me in the midst of the storm.

I remember the decision to hold on. When I made that choice, all that I grasped had to be redefined, redirected, reconstructed, and reconciled. Then, all that I clung to in the storm had to be released. As I learned to release, by simply letting go of the life I so wished to embrace, I demonstrated an enormous level of faith, power, and self-esteem—God-esteem!

Today is my birthday. I am celebrating life. But even in the joy of my celebration, I continue to struggle.

I feel the Father leading me to write about the winter. But I still have many doubts and questions. How can I share my pilgrimage of surviving devastation when I continue to fight some of the same battles as before? I still feel pain, uncertainties, insecurities, and unanswered questions. Life remains a mystery. Yet, I know that some of the most wonderful truths in life are mysteries. Have I really overcome? Am I a conquerer? If so, what have I defeated?

I do not always have answers. Maybe I no longer need them. To know the answers would shift my focus from the Father whom I desperately seek to follow, to myself, still full of limitations.

I have chosen to follow His leadership. I will write. But I need to share two things. First, my experience with pain is not past tense. The winter's wind continues to blow at times. But, so goes the flight! The flight to higher peaks comes in proportion to the valleys I have so intimately explored with you. Who am

I to determine the end of my flight? Perhaps I shall never arrive. I may only travel. Perhaps the way in which I travel will measure if I have truly survived, conquered, or arrived. Yes, I am more than a conqueror through Jesus Christ. My journey is simply to live now, for now is the only time there is. Second, my experience with pain is simply *my* experience. I remember thinking that I could not share my pain with anyone. *No one could ever understand the agony I had gone through,* I thought. Yes, that statement is true, but there is more. Pain is personal. No words can adequately describe anyone's pain. But pain is also universal. We all experience it at some time and in some way. What I can share is how I handled my pain and how I chose to grow through it.

Today is my birthday. Yet, everyday is. My gift to you today is my willingness to celebrate the storms of my life. This is not a story of a life relieved from pain, but a life joyfully lived through it. Maybe you can join me in celebrating a life that is transformed through winter.

I love you!

Marsha

Part I
The Fall
A Time to Die

Camouflaged Misery
Humility Enhanced
Please! Do Not Touch

I look into the mirror
Unsure of who I see
It is not You
But it is not me
Who is it that feels this misery?

I feel so sick, Father
As I remember my life
Claiming to be strong
When I know all along that who I am
And what I seek will never last.

I have spent my life so foolishly
Seeking things that cannot last

I could have changed the world
But now, is it really too late?

This is the life of camouflaged misery
I've smiled to make them think I am happy
My life has been spent trying to find a way
To satisfy this hunger in my soul
Somewhere I got lost in the crowd
I am small, I have run out of control.

If only I could have one other day
My life would be Your own
Though the world may think me strange
I will speak only of Your name
My life will be sincerely Yours.

As I lay my pen aside
I humbly lay myself down
Please! Crucify my pride
For as long as I have breath to breathe
I will speak Your name to every soul in need
Together, we will be freed
From our own misery.

—Marsha Spradlin

1
Camouflaged Misery

When I hoped for good, evil came;
when I looked for light, then came darkness.
The churning inside me never stops;
days of suffering confront me
(Job 30:26-27).

July 1983

The traffic in North Dallas was always congested—regardless of the time of day, and this day was particularly bothersome. The freeway between my office and condominium appeared to be more of a parking lot than an interstate highway. Barbara and I were agitated. We had left work early to get an edge on the traffic and the journey toward an overdue vacation.

Eventually, we managed to maneuver through the multilanes to an alternate route. The moment we arrived at the condominium complex where we each lived was the moment this energetic duo changed roles. We quickly came out of our suits and heels and slipped into T-shirts, jeans, and tennis shoes. We exchanged our briefcases for suitcases, released feelings of stress and tension, and breathed in that "Ah! Vacation-at-last" feeling.

Barbara made the sandwiches while I strapped our bicycles on the back of my Toyota. In less than forty-five minutes after arriving home, we were sunshine-bound—headed east on Interstate 20 on a twelve-hour marathon drive to Gulf Shores, Alabama. Gulf Shores was the vacation choice of the Spradlin family. When I was a child, our family enjoyed many vacations there. This week would be no exception. I could hardly wait to share this special place with Barbara, my dearest friend.

The drive was long, hard, and tiring. After all, we had already put in a full day at the office. Yet, we savored each moment. Even though Barbara and I lived in the same building, worked in adjacent offices, and even attended the same church, we seldom had time simply to visit. I loved this friend. She was perhaps the only person in my life with whom I felt completely safe. We had shared our fears, joys, fantasies, and even our dreads. She knew me well. Our friendship was a gift from the good and perfect Giver. It was rich, significant.

We certainly proved true the theory that time goes faster when you're having fun. The seven vacation days quickly escaped. How could we have packed so much into what felt like a long weekend?

I could best describe our week as an aesthetic experience. Sunrises painted the morning sky with brilliant reds and purples. My ears tickled as the ocean clapped the white beach rhythmically with its splashing salty waves. It was enchanting, soothing, and peaceful. It was no effort to relax.

Barbara, Mother, Daddy, and I walked on the beach early to watch the sunrise. We bicycled down the coast, chased tennis balls, cooked hamburgers, ate frozen yogurt, played Monopoly, and jogged after dark. Daddy always won and was furious when I tried to cheat!

I wanted to savor the week and file it away in my permanent memory of happiness and joy. It made a formative impression on my soul—the calm before the storm perhaps.

The time came to say good-bye to Mother and Daddy. They had become family to Barbara, too. Good-bye is never easy for our close family. After hugs and kisses, and Daddy checking my oil for the third time, we headed west—followed by two dirty bicycles. The drive seemed slower. Neither Barbara nor I seemed to have the enthusiasm or motivation to simply drive. We found many excuses to stop. The long and exhausting trip was fragmented with moments of depression. Neither of us were looking forward to reentry. Barbara and I both agreed that anything accomplished our first day back in the office was merely coincidental.

Life, for me, was full of pressure. Each moment was survival. Demanding as it was, I had a wonderful job. Being a state consultant for the world's largest Protestant denomination called for more commitment than many professions combined. My position required a great deal of travel—mostly in Texas. It insisted on creativity and an enormous amount of energy. For me, it was perfect. But like all jobs, it, too, had its own unique set of hazards. I lived under the constant strain of feeling the need to be all things to all people at all times.

We made the drive home less monotonous by listening to cassette tapes and singing along. Barbara found, embedded in the cassette box in the back seat, an old tape of "Leaning on the Everlasting Arms." I shall always remember singing it at least a dozen times—changing parts and singing louder each time. The rich truths running through the melody of that old song sank deep into my soul:

> What a fellowship, what a joy divine,
> Leaning on the everlasting arms;
> What a blessedness, what a peace is mine,
> Leaning on the everlasting arms.
>
> Leaning, leaning,
> Safe and secure from all alarms;
> Leaning, leaning,
> Leaning on the everlasting arms.
>
> Oh, how sweet to walk in this pilgrim way,
> Leaning on the everlasting arms;
> Oh, how bright the path grows from day to day,
> Leaning on the everlasting arms.
>
> What have I to dread, what have I to fear,
> Leaning on the everlasting arms?

I have blessed peace with my Lord so near,
Leaning on the everlasting arms.

My vacillation with depression was interrupted about one hour before we reached the Texas line. Barbara was driving. I had been asleep. I woke up suddenly to find a strange rash sprinkled on the upper portion of my left leg. *Maybe I had a little too much sun,* I thought. Or, maybe it is an allergic reaction to fun! I felt a pinch of concern, yet quickly chased it away.

We arrived home around 9:00 PM. After unloading the bikes and suitcases and dumping at least half of the Gulf of Mexico's sand out of my shoes and car, I decided that my tired muscles deserved some excitement. Jogging had become a form of therapy for me. So, I slipped into my running shoes, warmed up, and set out for a forty-five-minute run. After only five minutes, I felt like a sponge. I could not lift my left leg. My arms began to tingle, and my efforts to breathe were more like grasping for air. But I was determined to make at least one mile.

No way! My competitive nature suddenly gave in. Slowly, I climbed the three flights of stairs feeling defeated and extremely exhausted. I opened the door and quickly sank onto the couch—the first available place. Barb called moments later. Getting up to answer the phone was tough, but I did.

"Hey, you're back early!"

I couldn't admit that I couldn't run a mile so I simply backed out of the conversation by changing the subject. I could hardly stay awake to finish talking. All I wanted to do was sleep.

At 2:30 AM, I awoke. I had gone to sleep on the couch. Inside I heard those familiar tapes of Mother saying, "Marsha, put on your pajamas and get into your bed. You know better than to sleep in your clothes." Such guilt! I slowly managed to get to the bathroom. There I discovered a large lump on the right side of my neck. My face was pale, my vision blurred, and I suddenly felt overwhelmed with a tingling pain. *Aspirin,* I thought. *This calls for two aspirin and a hot bath.*

Morning came earlier than usual. Perhaps I slept fast. The phone rang at 7:00 AM. It was my friendly wake-up call. Barb knew of my tendency to oversleep. Getting me on my feet was always a challenge for her. The moment I tried to say hello, we both knew I had it.

"Marsh, you've got a bug. You had better call the office and let them know you're not coming in today."

"Sick? Not me! I simply won't allow myself to give in to something so silly. I don't have the time or the patience to deal with this, Barb."

For me, illness was something everyone else had to deal with. Not me. I had no respect for illness. In fact, sick people got on my nerves. In my opinion, most illness was simply a plea for attention. Besides, I could not call in sick after a week of rest and relaxation. How embarrassing!

My attitude toward illness was justified, I felt. I had grown up in a three-parent home: Mother, Daddy, and Mama Amy— my maternal grandmother and very best friend. Mama Amy was always suffering from something. She never left the house without her little navy blue suitcase full of medicines, cure-alls, potions, secret remedies, and ointments. I never really minded that; after all, she was Mama Amy—my special friend. What I did mind was the way people made fun of her and her little blue medicine bag. Whether or not her ailments were real or in her head, I was convinced that her chronic condition was real to her. I remember being angry when family members and friends made fun of her. Maybe that is why I promised myself as a young child that I would never be sick, and I would never carry a navy blue suitcase. So far, I had kept most of that promise. I had never owned a navy blue suitcase, and when-ever I was sick, I simply denied it and kept it concealed.

Three days lapsed before I was alert enough to care. I agreed to call Dr. Kennedy, my regular physician, only because of Barbara's pressure. It came in the form of obligation. She had fixed soup, juice, and even picked up the slack at the office.

Dr. Kennedy was out of the office, so I agreed to go to a hospital emergency room. Barbara offered to take me, but my self-sufficiency won. I drove myself and waited alone for two hours. I preferred it that way.

I began to think that perhaps I was suffering from amnesia. Since they had not called my name, I felt I must have forgotten it. Ah, at last!

"Miss Spradlin!"

I stepped on the scales to start the routine evaluation. There was nothing routine about the results. I had lost seven pounds in just a week. *Hospital scales are usually wrong,* I thought. Forty-five minutes later, a tall, skinny doctor pulled the curtain in my examination corner.

"I'm Dr. Hill. What seems to be the problem?"

"I am really fine, I think. I just came in to please my friends." Dr. Hill ordered a complete lab exam including X rays, blood work, and cultures. My suntanned legs dangled off the side of the examination table. I felt more anxiety with each moment of waiting. I was concerned not that he would find anything new, but that what he found would relate to a preexisting problem: one carefully concealed.

Eight years earlier, I had been diagnosed with a disease that was tubercular in nature—systemic sarcoidosis. The symptoms are much like those of lupus or even tuberculosis. A systemic disease can spread and go in and out of remission. I had it in my lungs and probably lymph glands. I knew far more already about doctors, X rays, and biopsies than most people learn in a lifetime. My disease had been in remission for several years. That was good since treatment was usually not effective. If I lost my remission status, the disease would spread to other organs, joints, and even to my skin and eyes. I feared not only the devastation of the disease but also the thought of "going public" if I had to be treated.

Dr. Hill was gone for a while, and his quick appearance again frightened me. "Young lady, you are sick!"

This statement describing my condition was almost funny, but I was too sluggish even to laugh. One shot and two X rays later, Dr. Hill scratched his head and said, "It could be strep throat, a virus, or mononucleosis. We will know when the tests come back next week. Meanwhile, I have a couple of questions for you."

He stuck two chest X rays on a screen and used his pencil to circle half a dozen tumors inside my lungs. "These appear to be tubercular," he said.

"A slight detail omitted on my part. I should have mentioned it before the X rays. I have systemic sarcoidosis. I am in remission. At least, I hope so."

"That is what concerns me. Tell me about the last few days."

"Besides losing weight, I have had trouble walking, and my joints are stiff. I ache. I feel I have fever. I can't breathe, but that is not unusual. My vision has been blurred."

"Marsha, these are all symptoms of active systemic sarcoidosis. I am going to order additional blood tests which usually indicate the activity level. Meanwhile, I think we should be positive and assume you have a virus. I am sending the cultures to the lab. But I'm concerned about the knots in your abdomen and neck. I want you to start these antibiotics immediately and call Dr. Kennedy. He is a good doctor, Marsha. I want him to do a complete follow-up. I will call him as soon as we have the results of these tests today. For now, go home. Rest and eat!"

I drove home feeling a familiar concern. I had every reason to be concerned. I had been a master at hiding this disease. In fact, while applying for graduate school a few years earlier, I went to a walk-in clinic that was famous for simply asking, "Are you in good health?" If the answer was yes, the staff signed the appropriate papers without tests or X rays.

This disease was diagnosed the summer after my college graduation. Strangely enough, it happened only weeks after Mama Amy died. So far, I had been very lucky. But that did not mean my family had not experienced fear and frustration. They feared the potential consequences of the disease. They knew that it could spread next to the liver or even the heart. Then my eyes and joints could be affected. Blindness and death were also possibilities, but that happened rarely and to other people. Not me.

I got home just in time to answer the telephone. Dr. Kennedy had already called in from out of town and received Dr. Hill's message. "I want to see you tomorrow."

Leave it to me to find an excuse. I did not see Dr. Kennedy for two weeks. Not knowing was easier than knowing. By the end of those two weeks I had improved a lot. The swelling had gone down, and my energy level had gone up. I felt ridiculous seeing a doctor when I felt fine, but I finally gave in.

Dr. Kennedy had a reputation as one of Dallas's finest young physicians. I simply adored him. He reminded me of a teddy bear. He wasn't much older than I was, and his dimples and boyish mannerisms made me laugh. I had complete trust in him as a physician and friend.

His exam revealed absolutely nothing. Somehow, the lab report from Dr. Hill had been lost in the mail. Dr. Kennedy had nothing with which to verify the information from Dr. Hill. The only thing he knew was that I had lost four more pounds. My once 130-pound body was now down to 119.

"You're getting a little on the thin side, Marsha. For a 5'7" frame, I would suggest you put on about five pounds. You need a little extra cushion that most of us can do without. I want you to spend the next two weeks resting and eating," he instructed; then he instantly covered his ears. He knew I was getting ready to rebound with excuses. Smiling, with his hands on both sides of his face, he backed out of the door.

"See you in two weeks."

Summer was usually busy where I worked. We were only two weeks away from our state leadership conference in which we trained 2,000 women. I knew that when I returned to work,

I would not only find my office embedded with paper work, projects, and telephone messages, but with a state leadership training event coming up as well. It would be easier to resign and start over in a month than dig out of this. But the pile of work did help redirect my attention away from myself and the "what ifs" that had been infiltrating my thoughts.

Each morning, before stepping into the shower, I was startled at my reflection in the full-length mirror in the bathroom. My clothes began to feel like they were falling off. My face seemed shallow, and my skin loose. *Where is the weight going?* I wondered. I had never focused on my weight before; I never needed to. But now was different. I bought a pair of inexpensive scales. Deep inside, I knew I had better start paying more attention to this.

The August heat convinced me that I needed to wear the coolest clothing I could find to the leadership conference in Waco. As I tried on outfits to decide what to take with me, I realized I had nothing to wear. This was a perfect reason to shop. However, I had never needed an excuse.

Barbara and I swung by our favorite dress shop one evening after work. I had been a size ten. We agreed that an eight should be perfect. We were both wrong. A six was a little loose! As I tried on clothes, I read concern in Barbara's eyes.

"Shouldn't you call Dr. Kennedy, Marsha?"

My reflection in the tiny room of mirrors convinced me. "I promise, Barb, but let's wait until after Waco. You know how much we'll eat there. Maybe I simply haven't been eating enough."

Deep inside, I knew I was camouflaging my misery. I knew I was sick, but I continued to wonder who could comfort my fears and dry the tears that no one could see. I felt caught like a leaf in the wind. I could not grasp all that was happening.

The meeting at Waco was its usual success. I was prepared for my assignments—but just barely. But I was not prepared for the many comments about my appearance from the participants. Dozens of well-meaning, motherly types expressed concern in the most inappropriate ways:

"You look awful."

One woman even asked Barbara if I was anorexic. Neither of us was familiar with that disease. We decided it must be some kind of virus.

The more people focused their attention on my body, the more I withdrew. Withdrawal was all I knew to do to protect myself from the interrogation and being associated with illness. I worked hard to conceal my concern about myself. I simply refused to recognize my physical decline.

Weeks translated into months. As each day escaped, so did my energy and zeal for life. I was deeply aware that something serious was wrong, and I was beginning to live a fragmented life. My fear intensified as I realized I could no longer hide the fact that I was ill. In late October, Dr. Kennedy called: "Just checking up on you, Marsha."

I felt a touch of anger. He was making such a big deal out of this. Yet, I was comforted that he was still interested.

"I'm fine. Busy, but fine."

"Have you continued to lose?"

"Maybe a little."

"I want to see you. I think it is time we do a complete series of tests. I may want you to see Dr. Johnson. He is a gastrointestinal man. He may be able to see something I have not picked up."

"I simply do not have time right now, Dr. Kennedy. Fall training is coming up. I have a full itinerary already."

"Humor me, Marsha."

On the next Monday, I spent at least twenty minutes driving in circles looking for a parking place at the medical center where Dr. Kennedy practiced. The parking lot ordeal was not nearly as complex as the one that was to come.

Dr. Kennedy had ordered a long succession of tests. The thumping, probing, sticking, listening, waiting, absorbed not

one day . . . but months. X rays, electrocardiograms, encephalo-
grams, spinal taps, brain waves, body scans, gastroscopic
probes, biopsies, and endless green machinery infiltrated my
life.

The "what-if" syndrome began to dominate my thoughts. I
imagined the worst, but of course communicated to others that
I was not concerned. On one occasion, Dr. Kennedy asked me
to call him to get some test results. I decided not to call. *If he
wants me to know something, he will tell me,* I thought. He did.

"Marsha, sorry for not calling sooner, but I wanted another
specialist to look at your films. We agree that more tests are
needed. You have all indications of malabsorption syndrome.
That means your body does not absorb nutrients. There can be
a hundred reasons for this. Some can be fixed quickly. Some
are certainly more devastating. We feel that the systemic sarcoidosis is not active right now, but we are concerned that the
stress of the weight loss could throw you out of remission.
Let's see. This is nearly Thanksgiving weekend. What if we
scheduled you for, say, first thing Monday morning? Go home.
Eat plenty of turkey and goodies, and I will arrange for a
biopsy."

"Biopsy? Who said anything about a biopsy? I have had
enough of those already."

"Marsha, we have to know. It's not that painful. In fact, I
will arrange for you to be asleep. Now go home and enjoy the
holiday."

I felt anger building. I was on a treadmill and unable to get
off; I was unwilling to accept what I knew. I was sick, very sick
and needed help—but I continued to reject it. Even though the
sun was shining outside, I felt the chill of winter creeping in.

Reflections on Perfectionism

I always secretly wished for perfectionism—wanting to rise
above my own human inadequacies. My solution for enduring
weakness was simply to ignore or deny my limitations. By

doing so, others were likewise convinced. It did work. Often people would comment, "Are you ever weak?"

If it is true that we learn from weakness, we grow in direct proportion to the amount of lack and limitation we recognize. If we refuse to recognize weakness by simply ignoring it, we refuse to recognize our ability to rise above it through the resource of Jesus Christ.

He allows us to learn from failure, weakness, and pain. God does not expect us to change every inadequacy into strength but to learn from them. Lack and limitation can help polish our potential if we allow God to do the polishing.

I made several mistakes before I learned this. My first mistake was denial. I refused to admit that I was weak.

My second mistake was looking ahead and praying for things to be different. This wasted precious moments of life. *Now* is the only time there is.

My third mistake was also denial. I refused to recognize my Source of help. I would not acknowledge my Father's ability to know intimately my deepest thoughts and identify with my deepest feelings.

But after I made these mistakes, I learned something: It is the *process* of living through inadequacies, not the *elimination* of them, that pleases our Father. Freedom comes in applying God's plan, not eliminating life's pain.

My most valuable lessons and spiritual growth happen while I am in the middle of the storm. My pain is not a barrier but a vehicle toward victory. Today!

Our love was some kind of magic
It eased the pain
And filled the void of our lives
With patience, kindness, and truth.

I could search the whole world over, I thought
And never find one as loving and true
We must be a part of His tapestry.
Our souls bonded together like a metal alloy.

How quickly love can change
How could our love be so broken?
Whose fault is it?
Someone is to blame
Was I looking for Your love in all the wrong places
I know I shall never know love again
Until I find perfect love in You.

I now walk on the edge of disaster
I do not have the skill to make it through
My humility is enhanced
As I sit alone cold and mystified.

Can You heal my broken heart?
I am lost in indecision
I need You, Father, to take me by the hand
Show me the way to set my sights on things above
And on my way back home
Let me get lost in the strength of Your love.

I had never felt love like this before
Until I met You
I had never known a song so brilliant to sing
I have never known a friend could be so true
Until I found the joy in loving You.

—Marsha Spradlin

2
Humility Enhanced

For it is commendable if a man bears up
under the pain of unjust suffering
because he is conscious of God.
But how is it to your credit
if you receive a beating for doing wrong and endure it?
But if you suffer for doing good and you endure it,
this is commendable before God.
To this you were called, because Christ suffered for you,
leaving you an example,
that you should follow in his steps
(1 Pet. 2:19-22).

November 1983

Fall is a season of change. In North Texas, the changes of fall
are more subtle than they are in other places. Few amber and
gold leaves drop from trees. In fact, there are few trees! People
in that part of Texas have to look to things other than nature
to signal the changes of fall—football, for example, and particularly the Dallas Cowboys.

I found waiting in checkout lines—and other public places,
for that matter—more entertaining in the fall. People everywhere would enter into a commentary on how "our" boys
were doing.

For me, the changes of fall were more drastic and personal.
As the trees released their few leaves, making way for new life,
my body escaped. Slowly, yet consistently. In nature, the or-
ganic process makes way for new life. Little did I know that
the mysterious process inside my body was also preparing me
for a new life. But just as the trees remain dormant for a while,
I, too, was about to enter my own state of silence.

On Tuesday before Thanksgiving, I flew to Mobile, Alabama, to celebrate with my family. Holidays were always special for us. Our customs and traditions were simple. Each year
my sister and brother and their families and I would gather at

our parents' home for the feast. Like mothers everywhere, mine cooked for days.

This was a special year. Jeff, someone special to me, was to arrive early Wednesday morning for the holiday. He usually came for Christmas and other special events. I could hardly wait. It had been a couple of months since we were together. We both had had a busy fall, and time with Jeff was long overdue.

I met Jeff while in graduate school in Texas. We sat next to each other in a philosophy class. *S's* always sat next to each other: Saunders and Spradlin. By midsemester, we decided it would be easier and much more fun to struggle together than apart. We started studying together several times each week. Jeff was much smarter than I—especially in philosophy. I can think of no better way than discussing philosophy to get thoroughly acquainted with someone: What is knowledge? What is beauty? What is the meaning of logic? The challenge of existentialism? What is real? Occasionally, we discussed more important things (!) like birthdays, hobbies, favorite movies, colors, and foods.

This sandy, blond-haired young man was my description of a gentleman. I enjoyed Jeff. His eyes communicated enormous trust and peace. Our relationship grew to the point that we were more than study buddies. Jeff Saunders became my best friend. We spent our free time on picnics in the park, driving in the country, fishing, walking in the woods, and simply sitting together and saying nothing. There was no question that we loved each other; the remarkable thing was how much we liked each other, too.

After graduation, we took jobs in different states, but our friendship remained a priority. We sought opportunities to be together. He was handy to have around, especially when I needed something fixed. He was an engineer by profession and an entrepreneur by personality. In my opinion, Jeff Saunders could do almost anything.

Jeff was aware of my illness. I did not want him to be startled when he saw me. He had expressed a great deal of compassion and concern. But, more than anything else, he had shown how much he cared beyond how I looked. He was one of the few men in my life whom I honestly felt enjoyed me for who I was instead of my appearance. Our relationship certainly had normal human physical tendencies, yet I never felt abused by Jeff or threatened by him. We were friends—the kind of friends who enjoyed the simplicity of just being friends. We certainly had not planned to care deeply. It was good, refreshing, and gratifying.

Preparing to meet Jeff's plane was an ordeal. I tried to find a loose sweater to hide my emaciated body. I knew Jeff would accept me, but I was not totally sure I did. Frustrated and concerned, I simply covered myself with the only sweater that looked decent.

Rushing to the airport turned out to be useless. Jeff's plane had been delayed in Atlanta due to fog. I had to wait at least an hour before he arrived. I was already nervous. The delay only intensified my feelings. I could not wait to see Jeff, but I feared he would reject me. I was not the woman he remembered from school—much less a few months ago.

I had begun to resemble one of those starving children on another continent. My weight had dropped about three more pounds since my recent appointment with Dr. Kennedy. As each pound left me, my positive concept, outlook, and attitude likewise escaped. I guess I was learning lessons in self-respect. But, at that time, I would have denied ever linking my good with what I looked like, where I was, and who I was with.

Finally, I heard the announcement that Jeff's plane had arrived. I mingled into the crowd of people eager to receive friends or loved ones for the holidays. I felt a nervous flutter that intensified as each person entered the waiting area. Each face stimulated conflicting feelings. I was relieved it was not

Jeff, but I was also disappointed because I so much wanted to see him.

Those thoughts and feelings left me the moment Jeff walked through the gate. I simply embraced him. If he was startled at my appearance, he certainly hid it well. We hugged for what seemed to be ten minutes and laughed. "Really, Jeff, don't you think folks are staring?"

"I don't care; they are simply jealous!" Jeff wrapped my tiny hands around a small gift he had protected during the bumpy flight from Atlanta: a red rose.

He said nothing about how I looked. *Maybe I am making too big a deal out of this,* I thought.

Thanksgiving morning finally arrived. I had set my clock early, so I could prepare my traditional Thanksgiving breakfast feast. I was not exactly the world's greatest cook, but I did enjoy banging around in the kitchen on occasion. The men especially enjoyed this tradition because it would be hours before our celebration of turkey and trimmings. Soon after I went into the kitchen, Jeff must have heard me drop something and joined me. We played more than cooked. We were more like two teenagers than a couple of young professionals. It didn't matter what we were doing as long as we were doing it together.

We spent the day walking, sitting in the swing, washing my car, and installing cruise control, and sneaking little pieces of turkey and fudge from the kitchen. Still, he had not spoken one word about my emaciated physical condition.

Late afternoon brought nephews, nieces, and other family members. This was a special day, and I was glad Jeff was there to share it. Only one month earlier, my fifteen-month-old nephew Justin had suffered a life-threatening illness. He spent over three weeks in intensive care with complete kidney failure. Physicians worked around the clock to identify the cause, but we had no answers. We had come within moments of losing our precious little one. Just as we had no explanation for

his close call with death, we had no explanation for his survival
—except that it was a miracle.

Jeff was crazy about "my kids." They, too, enjoyed "Uncle
Jeff." I was always a little amazed at how well Jeff related to
the little ones. It was as if he had children of his own. They
were as comfortable with him as each member of my family
was. While Jeff entertained the gregarious kids, my sister Teresa and I escaped for a brisk walk.

"Marsha, I think Jeff's in love."

"Absolutely not! We are friends, Teresa. That is the way we
like it. He has his life, and I have mine. If we were in love, that
would mess it up."

"You just wait, Sis. You have all of the symptoms of being
bitten. I predict that you and Jeff will be married by this time
next year."

"I promise, you will be one of the first to know. But don't
hold your breath."

Teresa was only one year older but had strong instincts. She
did not often give me advice, but when she did, she was strong
in her opinion and delivery. She was absolutely certain Jeff and
I were made for one another. While I verbally disagreed, inter-
nally I could not have been more certain she was right. Maybe
I wasn't ill after all. Perhaps I had just been bitten by a Saunders bug!

Jeff was scheduled to depart for Atlanta on Saturday night.
Once he checked his baggage and received his boarding pass,
we found a quiet corner. Only then did we talk about me and
the uncertainties.

"Marsha, I love you. In fact, I can't seem to get my mind on
anything else. I do not know what I would do if something
happened to you. You know what I am saying, don't you? You
must know that I think you are beautiful just like you are. My
love for you is stronger than an attachment to your body. I am
here for you, kid. I am fighting for you and for us. I want you
to feel free to let me be here for you."

We tightly squeezed each other's hands as we cried together. I was unable to say anything. We hugged tightly, kissed, and he was gone.

As Jeff's plane lifted off, my spirit sank. How could this be happening? How could I be losing myself at the exact time I felt I had found secure love?

I did not drive directly home. Instead, I circled the city a couple of times. I remembered the "old" days when I used to live in Mobile, the days before Jeff, before the illness. The days of high school football games and friends. The days of no worries—just the hopes of the future. Where were those days? Would life ever be easy again?

On Sunday morning, I flew back to Dallas. I had traveled on that flight many times. I enjoyed using the headphones of my cassette player to listen to my favorite classical music. I needed the solitude, the retreat, the time to think.

While I knew that many fears and uncertainties were building inside, I still felt a strong element of hope: Jeff. I recognized that my love for him was far more than friendship. That was frightening, but it was also exhilarating. He added stability.

On Monday morning, I arrived at the medical center early, following through with Dr. Kennedy's request for additional tests and a biopsy. Barbara was convinced that I could not go alone. While I preferred to solo this ordeal, Barbara's presence was fine. I filled out multicopies of forms granting permission for them to perform the biopsy. Suddenly, I heard my name.

"I have been looking everywhere for you. I am so glad to find you since I have to hurry to the office. Folks are wanting a full report. I told them I would just drop by on my way in."

I was mortified. I was angry. What right did Anna have to pry into my private world? Anna was a friend from work, yet not the type of friend to whom I chose to reveal my inner private world. At this point, I did not want exposure. I did not need support—just protection. She was a friend, but she was neither Jeff nor Barbara. Even though I felt my anger intensely,

I did not want to communicate hostility. But I did make it clear she was not to report anything at the office. I would share anything anyone needed to know.

I felt horrible because I overreacted toward Anna. She had simply wanted to express her love and concern, but I had rejected her.

The biopsy procedure went fine. I remember very little because of the sedatives. But I do remember my pastor and Barbara each standing on opposite sides of the bed in the recovery room. I loved my pastor. I wasn't sure how he learned about the biopsy, but I was glad he was there. The sedative lessened my need for privacy, I guess.

Dr. Kennedy came by before discharging me and said, "It will be a few days before we know the results. Meanwhile, I have scheduled additional tests for nearly every day of the following two weeks."

December 1983
Over the next weeks, I was stuck, poked, X-rayed, questioned, and basically humiliated. I felt abused by the endless tests, questions, and exposure to high doses of X ray. So far, we knew I had malabsorption syndrome, but we did not know the cause.

My world began to sink. Barbara and Jeff were the only two, besides family, with whom I shared my feelings.

As the weeks passed, I noticed an incredible sense of atrophy. My muscles were dying, it seemed. I felt intense pain and could find no relief. Even sleeping became difficult. I was unable to lie in bed very long without feeling enormous pain due to my lack of body tissue. I could not even walk from room to room without having to stop. I often sat in the car and cried because I dreaded climbing the stairs at my condo.

Perhaps the strongest indication that I was giving in to the illness was my lack of interest in anything—even myself. I had always taken a great deal of pride in my grooming and physical appearance. My hair had to be perfect and my makeup exact. As my weight dropped into the lower nineties, I did not have the energy to do anything about my appearance, nor did I feel that it mattered.

By mid-December, I was a walking cavity of concern for everyone. Even people who had never seen me before stopped and stared. I wanted to hide from the abuse I felt from people's comments and lack of sensitivity. I just wanted to sleep. Dr. Kennedy grounded me from all work and professional engagements. "No travel, Marsha, until we get this thing figured out and corrected," he said. "If you have not improved by January, I'm checking you into the hospital. You could drop dead if you continue this decline."

I remember very little about Christmas. I flew home because Mother was horrified by the very thought of my driving. I basically felt like a zombie. I had little to say, but I felt things very deeply.

The main thing I do remember about Christmas was that Jeff was there. He had just returned from a month-long business trip to India. He brought gifts of Indian rugs, rings, and other goodies. I remember sitting in the den and trying to stay alert while he told of his adventures and showed hundreds of slides. I listened as I sat wrapped in a blanket to stay warm. Then I cried because I could not get warm. Jeff rubbed my bony shoulder and just was there for me. We talked very little. I slept most of the time.

Jeff's presence was good for Mom and Dad. They—especially Dad—needed someone to talk to and lean on. Jeff and Dad were more like father and son than father and potential son-in-law. They took several walks together during those days. I knew their conversations were about me, but I did not have the energy to find out the details. My defense was down. I merely struggled to survive.

My emotions were extremely vulnerable. I would cry for no reason and become agitated at times. I thought I was going crazy because I could not stop crying. I remember feeling profound anger not directed at anyone or anything in particular. It would ignite instantly. Usually it was triggered because the TV was too loud or the room was too noisy. But the noise outside my body was not what was really making me angry; it was the noise inside that caused the agitation.

I felt my hurt was uniquely mine. I had a hard time believing that others had ever suffered this much. But as I continued to tell myself that it was not real, the fear continued to build. I saw it coming but could do nothing to keep it from being a part of my own community of pain.

While I never contemplated ending my life, I did develop a sympathetic understanding for those who do harbor such a dark impulse. I felt I could handle anything if I knew its name and nature. But I did not know how to handle the unknown.

Mother protected me from the crowds of concerned friends who wanted to stop by to see what I looked like. She screened my calls and ran interference. My brother was unable to say anything without almost losing his composure. On one occasion, he put his hand around my arm only to discover that his seven-year-old daughter's arm was far larger than that of his nearly thirty-year-old sister.

January 1984

I arrived back in Dallas during the second week of January. By that time, Dr. Kennedy discussed in-depth my tests with several of the experts. Together, they devised a strategy.

I had been on a high dosage of beta-blocker drugs for several months. The systemic sarcoidosis was not the only condition I had concealed. A heart condition had also tiptoed into my secret life. This condition was linked to a prenatal birth defect. It brought a full range of symptoms: migraine headaches, various levels of dehydration, extreme pain in joints, instant, unexplainable fatigue, tricky heart beats, numbness in arms and legs, and extremely low blood pressure. Because of the weight decline, my blood pressure had likewise declined. Beta-blocker drugs only made it worse. For that reason, the doctors decided to quickly pull me off all drug therapy.

Dr. Kennedy explained that because I might go into shock if my blood pressure got too low, there was no time for slow withdrawal.

That seemed simple, but it was one of the most painful experiences up to that point. I would never have considered myself a drug addict, but suddenly I was going through drug withdrawal.

The following days were like a nightmare. I felt like I had a high fever and a tension inside. I ached to the core. I trembled and was convinced I would not live through each new day, but the fact that I survived helped me know I could endure almost anything.

February 1984

During the following weeks, Jeff remained in close contact. He called at least twice a day. By late February, he couldn't stand it any longer. "I am coming to Dallas," he asserted. I really preferred that he not come, but I was too weak to tell him.

Jeff arrived for a weekend visit, and once again we recognized that we loved each other. This time Jeff announced his intentions to move to Dallas. I was thrilled.

Jeff spent part of his visit to Dallas looking for housing and talking to engineering firms. He was a brilliant engineer and had a successful career with a major industry. He had invented several pieces of equipment for manufacturing firms and had received several patents and awards. As a result, he had a strong financial base. He could afford me. While we did not publicly announce our intentions, we were serious about a permanent commitment.

Friday morning after breakfast, Jeff and I visited several jewelry stores. We quickly agreed on what we liked and did not like in rings. But I believe I would have been agreeable about any choice. I simply did not have the energy to stand for any length of time and discuss it. I seemed to have lost my ability to form an opinion.

Barbara and Jeff also had some time together. They were a support for each other as they focused their love, time, and energy toward helping me hold on to my frail hope.

Jeff was not scheduled to leave until Sunday morning. Saturday morning, I pulled together enough energy to prepare his favorite breakfast: an egg and cheese omelette with sausage. Afterwards, we moved to the living room, propped our feet on the coffee table, and sipped hot chocolate. Jeff's statement caught me off guard.

"Marsha, I must share something. I don't know really where to start, but before we go any further in our relationship, I must let you know about something in my background."

I began seeing red flags. *Watch out! He's about to throw a curve into your fantasy,* I thought.

"I have been married before, but we divorced shortly afterward. We were both very young. We made a mistake. Besides not having anything in common, neither of us were mature enough to make it work—but there is more."

Jeff reached into his back pocket and pulled pictures out of his wallet. Next to my picture was Kevin, his young son.

I was stunned, but compassion caved in. I wanted to hit him, yet hold him. My mind was unable to process exactly what he was telling me. I quickly dismissed it. Denial was my only defense.

"He looks just like you. I'm sorry, Jeff. That must've been awful and so painful for you." I could not believe my response was so full of mercy, love, and forgiveness. I must be sicker than I thought. Inside, I wanted to run, escape, scream. Outside, I simply hugged him and said nothing. We decided to make a good day out of the time we had left. But by midafternoon, darts and doubts had begun to rush in. I so much wanted and needed to trust Jeff, but I also wanted to be left alone. I found myself questioning everything he said. Finally, I announced that perhaps he should leave. I needed time to think. I needed time to adjust to what he had told me. I had to decide if I still loved him.

On Saturday night, I took Jeff to the airport early. I kissed him good-bye and drove away with a devastated spirit. My guard was strong until my car disappeared from his sight. I sank deeply into the steering wheel and cried from the deepest parts of my soul.

"God, what else can happen?" I screamed. "Where are you? What am I going to do with Jeff? He's the only good part of my life right now."

I could feel my spirit beginning to sink. I felt sick. I did not go home; instead, I drove for hours.

Barbara was out of town, and I did not want to be in my condo alone. It was decorated with Jeff's gifts and abilities. He had assembled every book case I owned. With his expert advice, we had hung my pictures. He was everywhere. It wasn't that I had lost him; I just wasn't sure I knew him. I realized his impact on my life. If I chose not to marry him because of the divorce, would I stick to my decision, or would I marry him because I was addicted to Jeff Saunders?

I got up early Sunday morning knowing what I had to do. Instead of dressing for Sunday School, I put a cold compress on my sore eyes. Picking up a note pad and pen, I carefully constructed my thoughts:

> Dear Jeff:
> You are charming, Jeff Saunders. I am addicted to you, I think. But I have strong feelings of doubt right now. I need time to think and find out for myself how much I really care. I guess I am now wondering if I love you or if I loved who I thought you were. Maybe I loved only who I wanted you to be for me.

I do not know. Please do not call; I will call you. Please love me
enough to give me time to know.
Love,
MARSHA

I rushed to the post office to mail the letter before I changed
my mind. Dr. Kennedy had given me a prescription for pain
as well as sleeping pills. It was not the physical pain that made
me so helpless but the desolate feeling of not having Jeff. I took
a couple pills and crawled into bed. I hoped I would wake up
to find out this was a dream.

Barb returned home late Monday night. She instantly knew
that one of two things were wrong—either I had received a bad
report from Dr. Kennedy or something had happened with Jeff.
I managed to get through the story. She was furious. She spent
the rest of the evening with me. In fact, she slept on the couch
that night. I was fragile physically as well as emotionally. Beth
recognized the intensity of my pain.

Late Tuesday night, I was ironing a shirt to wear to the
hospital the next day for more tests. The phone rang.

"Marsha? It's me, Jeff. We have a problem." Jeff spoke in a
quiet tone.

"You got my letter?" I asked.

"Not exactly."

Tears began to roll freely down my face. "I know we have
a problem, Jeff."

"No, there's more."

As soon as Jeff spoke, I heard someone in the background.
She took the phone. "Marsha, this is Linda. I'm Jeff's wife. Do
you hear a baby in the background? That's Kevin, our son. I
found your letter. I had suspected for some time that Jeff was
having an affair."

"No, not me. You've made a mistake. Jeff is divorced."

"I should know. I've been his wife for ten years. We've never
been separated, except for the times he's been away on busi-

ness trips. By the way, have you been spending holidays with my husband? I think he was with you when Kevin was born. I will see that you pay for this!"

Jeff grabbed the phone.

"Marsha! Linda found your letter. It is true, all of it."

"How could it be true? Jeff! Jeff! Speak to me."

He had dropped the telephone. I instantly hung up, ran into my bedroom, and buried myself in my pillow. I curled up as the pain pressed against my eyes. Barbara sat next to me on the bed and cried, "Dear, sweet friend! Why, God? Why is this happening to my friend? Hasn't she had enough?"

After an hour or so of spilling my soul to Barbara, she grabbed my coat and tightly wrapped it around me. I could hardly walk. Arm in arm, we slowly made it down the stairs. She tucked me inside her car, and we drove for hours saying nothing. We simply drove.

Words cannot describe what I felt. Barbara, too, was in misery. She loved Jeff. She, too, felt the humiliation of betrayal. As for me, the only hope I had now was the fear of holding on. Hold on to what? Will I ever love again? It is not worth the pain. I have never seen Jeff again.

March 1984

The tests scheduled for the morning after Jeff's call were postponed until later that week. Even though the storm was building inside, something within me continued to fight. It was the survival instinct, I guess. But I was still fighting with reality. I refused to accept that I could be only moments away from death. Barbara knew it. She had already rehearsed in her mind exactly what she would do in an emergency. She had memorized the phone number at the medical center. She was prepared.

We were only days away from my thirtieth birthday. The staff at my office had planned a party to surprise me and cheer me up after the crushing experience with Jeff. To demonstrate their love, they arranged for Mother to come for a visit. No one said anything about Jeff or my illness, but everyone was thinking the same thing: *This could be her last birthday.*

A thirtieth birthday is special, but few people have ever received the attention as this tiny person did for having lived thirty years. It was a special party complete with cake, candles, and decorations. My secretary had written a skit and performed it in full hilarious attire. It was a time of celebration, but the devastation never really left me. I felt compelled to appear "up" and to conceal my pain. I managed.

Mother stayed a couple of days after my birthday. Her birthday was the day after mine, so we celebrated again. I created havoc for her as I refused to acknowledge the seriousness of the illness. Dr. Kennedy had been wanting me to check into the hospital for weeks, but I refused. "Keep looking, Dr. K. You'll find it."

I now weighed eighty-six pounds. My spirit was fragmented. In secret, Mother managed to call Dr. Kennedy. He insisted that I go into the hospital the following week. I was unaware of the conversation.

On Saturday after my birthday, Mother flew home. She did not know she would be back in a couple of days. But she preferred to play along with my game rather than rock my shaky boat. Like all mothers, she wanted to stay. But this independent daughter refused to accept help or support. To accept it would be to accept the dreadful situation as real.

Just as he had promised Mother, Dr. Kennedy arranged for my hospitalization for the following Wednesday. As I sat in his office Monday afternoon, I pleaded, "Please, give me one more week. Let's see if this will turn around."

I did have the ability of persuasive speech. Somehow, I won.

Wednesday morning was harder than usual. I got up around 7:00 AM, only to discover that I now weighed eighty-two pounds. I simply went back into my bedroom, crawled under the covers, and slept until noon. I managed to get up with an appetite. I decided to heat up some leftovers for lunch. While I ate, I started to feel sick at my stomach. I put down my fork and walked over to the couch and crashed. Moments later, I heard a key in the lock. It was Barb. A surprise visit! "Hello, friend. What am I doing home? Well, I have a present." She placed into my hands a small package, wrapped in white with a tiny blue ribbon. "For you."

Tears flooded my eyes for no reason except that I loved her, trusted her, and needed her support. I opened the gift. Two little snowflake earrings. Perfect. It is so cold, Barbara. Will this winter ever be over?

Suddenly I felt a pounding inside my chest. I was overwhelmed with nausea.

"Barbara, I think I'm going to be sick."

I felt I would vomit. This was a new symptom. I had not done that since I was a preschooler. Barbara ran into the bathroom for wet towels. I got up quickly, trying to make it to the bathroom. As soon as I stood, I heard ringing inside my head. I felt hot coals burning my skin. The room was totally black. I could not see Barbara, I could not hear her. I could hear only the loud ringing noise inside my head. The pounding scared me. I was dying. I knew it. This is what it feels like. I screamed:

"Oh, please God. Not now. Can't You wait? Not now. Not now!"

Reflections on Wrong Assumptions

Until I got sick, I always secretly equated my worth with who I was with, what I looked like, or even where I was. All three were wrong assumptions. The fear of losing my body told me I was no longer good. The fear of losing my love, Jeff, whispered a message that I could only be happy when I was with him and loved by him.

Wrong assumptions? Perhaps one was that Jeff was perfect. He was not perfect. But as long as I needed him to be perfect, I risked feeling like a total failure for ever loving him. How could I have fallen for such a fake? How could I have been so misled? I began to feel rejected not only by Jeff but by God as well.

I wished I had known then that God does not love me because of what I do, who I am with, or even where I am. God loves me because absolute love is His nature.

Even deeper, though, I felt that God's love was measured by His blessing. He had blessed me with a strong body and a beautiful friendship. Now both were gone. Does that mean God no longer loved me? No. I am loved regardless of who I am with, what I look like, or what circumstances I find myself in. And you are, too.

It is late in the night
I am all alone
I sit like a stone or frightened child
Who darts away in fear.

I stare at the walls of disbelief
With eyes that cannot cry
Why does life have to be so sad
Will I ever heal?

I feel like an orphan
So I close my door
Leaving the world behind
Here I sit, all alone in my fortress
Seeking safety in the shelter of Your arms once more.

What I need is to be Yours again.
Who am I really living for?
Touch me, Father
With a vision that despises the things that do not please You
Take me back to the start
Create within me a new heart.

—MARSHA SPRADLIN

3
Please! Do Not Touch

If we die with him,
we will also live with him;
if we endure,
we will also reign with him
(2 Tim. 2:11).

March 13, 1984

My memory of March 13, 1984, is evasive and explosive—full of haunting shadows that dart forth when I least expect them. On command, I can recall the details. At other times, they flood forth because of some unknown impulse or stimulus. But in general, the details have simply escaped my ability to remember. My vision was stolen by pain. My ability to hear was overwhelmed by the loud ringing that echoed inside my entire body which was struggling to survive. It was torture and unlike any dying episode I had ever heard about or even read about in a science fiction book. It was like drowning. I was screaming for help! I wanted to swim, but no one could reach me. No one could throw me a lifeline. It was a painful dream—a nightmare.

* * * * * * * * * *

"What is your name? Can you hear me? Please try to tell me your name?"

The questions persisted, but I could think of no reason to respond. I thought the person speaking knew who I was. After all, he was my father.

Only moments before, he held me in his arms. *I must have fallen asleep during church,* I thought. That was not unusual for a little girl. On those occasions, Daddy would always wrap me in his strong arms and carry me quietly to the car. Once in the car, I was always semiawake.

During the ten-minute ride home, I wished we would never arrive. I simply wanted to sleep. Sleep meant rest. For an active nine-year-old, rest was easy.

"What is your name? Can you tell me who you are? Do you know where you are?"

Why so many questions? I thought. I knew exactly where we were—about three minutes from our house. I could tell because of the bumps in the road. Even though I thought I was asleep, I had counted each turn. The route was familiar. We had traveled those streets many times.

"What is your name? Please, try to wake up and tell me. If you can hear my voice, squeeze my hand."

This was not normal. Daddy never asked questions like this. He always let me sleep on the way home from church. I could not understand the questions. Why such interrogation? Even so, the sleep seemed sweeter, deeper, and more peaceful than any I had ever remembered. It was like a retreat or release. My Father's presence almost seemed to take my breath away.

Why doesn't Daddy turn up the heat? I am so cold, I thought. I never remembered being so cold before in my life; I didn't remember it being winter. *Will I ever be warm again?* But I was warm. I was confused. I was shivering outside, but I felt a warm glow inside. Even the glow was painful. I felt secure and warmth in God's presence.

"Marsha, wake up. We are moving you now. Try to wake up."

I always wanted to please Daddy. So, I tried. For a minute, it felt like a mistake. The moment I responded, the rest escaped, and the peace was gone. I was overcome with fear. The

warm. I wanted relief from the uncertainties that had consumed my life.

Reality came rushing in like a cold intruder. I knew what was
real. I was not nine years old. I was thirty. My father had not
carried me to the car because I had fallen asleep in church.
Instead, three paramedics had carried me down three flights of
stairs on a stretcher. They were so overwhelmed at the sight
of my emaciated body that they were afraid to touch me. The
vehicle was not a car. It was an ambulance escorted by three
fire trucks. The voice did not belong to my father but to one
of the three men who transported me from my condo to the
nearest hospital.

One impression was true. I never remembered winter being
so cold. I wondered if I would ever know the warmth of springtime again.

During the initial moments of my fight to stay alive, I struggled with reality and my semiconsciousness. I felt like I was
swimming. But I had no energy. Could no one help? Could no
one reach me? The only thing I was certain of was His presence. I felt His touch and heard Him whisper to hold on.

I spoke loudly to Him. I screamed out! "Not now. Please not
now!"

Only He heard me. No one observing the tragedy recalled
any sound or movement. While cold and fragile, I felt rays of
His holy light. My darkness was flooded with brightness as I
stood in the shadows of His magnificent love.

Only the powerful instinct to survive caused my body to
cooperate to bring back the life that was being sabotaged. The
struggle to stay alive was painful. In spite of the imprisonment,
the enslavement, the pain, my body continued to struggle to
choose life.

My mind grasped for reality. I thought of Barbara. I was
aware of her presence. I was unaware she had rehearsed for this
moment. She had memorized Dr. Kennedy's phone number.
She had known for some time that it was only days or mo-

ments until I would simply die or lose consciousness. But during those months, she had never voiced her pain. Her surprise visit was evidence of God's hand. She was there by divine appointment. I am convinced that all who entered my gates that day likewise had responded to the nudging of the Gentle Shepherd.

My first conscious memory was Barbara's voice. I felt confused. Someone was holding me. I could hear Barbara talking on the telephone from another room. I wondered with whom she was talking. The conversation sounded serious. Then I realized she was referring to me. I wanted to say, "Don't call Dr. Kennedy. I will be OK. I will wake up in a moment." But my voice was trapped inside my body which was not responding to anyone or anything. The confusion was reinforced as I realized that someone was holding me. How could she hold me and be in the other room? Ah! It was Pat from the office. Pat was holding me. How did she know to come?

Pat was gently stroking my head and holding my upper body tightly. She sat calmly on the floor whispering funny stories.

"Marsha, you are going to be fine, kid, but you have got to wake up for me. Look, Barb, I think she heard me."

Pat was not planning to come by that day. She simply felt "led" to come. When she arrived, I had been unconscious only twenty or thirty seconds. Barbara had not locked my front door. This was so unusual for her. We both were in the habit of always locking our doors. Shortly after coming in, Barbara opened the living room window for some fresh air.

When I lost consciousness, Pat was knocking at the door, identifying herself. Barb cried for help. With the window open, Pat quickly recognized Barb's voice. Because the door was unlocked, Pat was able to come in quickly. Both of these actions played a significant role in the chain of events that paved the way for my survival.

I guess if I could have chosen two people whom I did not mind seeing me that day, it would have been these two friends.

I remembered nothing about the several minutes that followed. But with each moment of consciousness, I remember enormous pain which knocked me out. I was in and out—mostly out. My next memory was hearing the sirens. The stomping of hurried feet up three flights of stairs communicated a sense of urgency. Once the paramedics arrived, I sensed they were simply standing, petrified at what they saw. *Why are they in such a hurry?* I wondered.

While I could not see them, I sensed the room was filled with men—all staring at my skeleton. I wanted to protect myself. I wanted to scream, "Please! Do not touch!"

There was obvious confusion about what to do. So, for moments, they stood watching me die. Barbara finally took charge and made the decisions. Later, we realized that no one expected me to live long enough to be transported to the hospital.

Barbara remained calm as she talked on the phone with the staff at the medical center. They insisted that I be transported immediately. But after talking with one paramedic who described my condition, they agreed I should not be transported across town to their facility. I would not have survived the trip. The paramedics decided they would move me immediately to the hospital across the street and contacted the emergency room which prepared for my arrival.

In my underwater state of consciousness, I remember hearing them talk. I knew they did not know what to do with me. I wanted to scream out again, but my voice was trapped inside.

"Please! Just pick me up and put me in the car. Either do something or get out and leave me alone!"

My next memory was the ride. I was not in Dallas mentally or emotionally. I had reverted to my childhood. I did wake up in the ambulance. Barbara was sitting next to me, smiling and holding my hand. The paramedics knew I was in shock. The constant interrogation was intended to arouse me in order to determine my degree of consciousness.

I have no memory of arriving at the hospital. My next conscious moment was inside the emergency room. Hot lights warmed my cold body. Someone draped me with a white sheet and several inches of blankets. Green curtains accented my feelings of being under water. People seemed to be in a hurry. An IV had been inserted and was already pumping fluids to my depleted body.

Apparently, I was suffering from shock as the normal defense systems were shutting down. This was complicated by a suspected cardiac arrest.

I could vaguely see an outline of a woman bent over me. While everyone seemed to be in a hurry, she seemed calm. I saw a gold snowflake swinging over my face. She was wearing a snowflake. I watched it swing back and forth in a rhythmic manner and tried to concentrate on it. I had to wake up, but being awake accented the pain I felt from the tubes and other devices. At that point, I had not received any sedatives to lessen the pain.

The snowflake. Is it winter? The snowflake was so beautiful. I felt almost in a trance as I watched it swing back and forth, just as I had swung back and forth in a cradle over my own grave.

I felt euphoria. I felt warm! I felt like I wanted to put my arms around this woman and tell her I loved her. I wanted her to hold me. Was she my mother? She seemed like my mother as she quietly cared for me. I wanted to tell her, "This is not really me. I am embarrassed that you are seeing me like this. I am more than this bag of bones. I am really sort of pretty, I think. I am smart. I have a job."

Then I realized I did not care if she ever knew who I was. Just like the snowflake, I was special, unique, not like anyone else. Just like the snowflake, I felt suspended in midair—floating. Hot tears streamed down my face.

Oh, don't let the snow melt. I thought. I felt wonderful. But I did not know why. I was not aware that I had received sedatives which were now starting to take affect. I felt only the euphoria of having gone on a trip—somewhere very special. I wanted to go home. I was still unsure if I was alive.

As the medications began to take effect and as the fluids replenished my thirsty body, I began to recognize voices. I heard Barbara. "Where is she? Someone get Barbara. I don't know where I am."

Barbara heard me, and in spite of the rule about not entering the trauma unit, she rushed in. Her comfort was incredible. She instantly put her hands over mine and pressed her cheek against my head.

"I don't remember coming here, Barb. What happened?"

"It's OK, Marsh! I think you're going to make it, now. Just hang on a little tighter."

"When they finish the test, can we go home?" I pleaded.

"I don't think so—not for some time, maybe. But let's not worry about that, OK?"

"Mother! Don't call her. Not yet. I think I'll get to go home, probably tonight. Don't call her. Please, tell me you won't call. She'll only worry."

Barbara was saved from making a promise she couldn't keep. The nurse swung back the curtains to prepare to start another IV.

"Honey, we are going to give you a little extra boost of this good stuff. You shouldn't feel anything."

"Why is everyone running around so hurried? Is somebody here bad sick?"

My nurse looked at Barbara as she said, "Yes, honey. Somebody here is really bad sick."

"Are they going to die?" I asked.

"We don't know. We are trying very hard to keep that from happening."

"Is there someone in here besides me?"

Barbara and my nurse both squeezed my hand.

"No, honey, you're the only patient we have right now. And you're keeping us plenty busy."

Within the hour, I could hear the physicians talking to Dr. Kennedy. Soon, one of them came in.

"As soon as you are a little more stable, Miss Spradlin, we're going to transport you to the medical center where Dr. Kennedy practices. They are much more able to deal with your case since they have all of your records."

A couple of hours passed. I must have slept most of that time. I knew something was going to happen when the paramedics began to gather. Once again, they stared. After they agreed on what they were to do, they gathered the equipment which weighed much more than the patient. IV bags, heart monitors, blood pressure cuffs all had to be organized. Then they just stood there. This time I simply said, "Pick me up and put me on that stretcher. I promise not to break. I'll walk if you don't hurry."

They laughed at my spunk which apparently broke the silence and sparked them to move.

I remember very little about this second trip. I do recall staring at the small silver screws in the ambulance ceiling. I counted them and wondered which way they screwed. Screws are brilliant. They hold things together. I remember forcing myself to think about those stupid screws; otherwise, I would have been forced to realize that I still might be dying.

It was nearly five o'clock. In all of my Dallas driving, I had never had such respect during peak driving hours. Cars responded to the sirens and quickly pulled aside. Since I could not see anything, Barbara kept me informed about our exact location. "Marsh, we are getting on the toll road. Hey, they're not making us pay the fifty cents. What a deal!"

Pat trailed right behind. It was an ordeal for her to try desperately to stay close in the traffic.

Again, my memory of arriving at the medical center escapes me. My next memory was being transferred into the intensive care emergency room. There Barbara stayed with me while the physicians looked at reports.

This was some place, not a curtain-type emergency room. It was medically sophisticated. Many bright lights hung from every angle. The room was large, but my elevated bed was in the center. A large clock was just above eye level. Even while Barbara stood over me, I stared at the clock. Time was escaping. It was slipping quickly. If I could only stop the hands on the clock. Nothing I could do would make it stop. I felt that if I could stop time, I would have a chance to survive.

If only they would turn off the bright lights, I thought. The brightness was not natural. But I could see! I had forgotten that I had not been able to see earlier. I wanted to sleep.

"Barbara, please don't call Mother. Not yet."

Barbara changed the subject. "Millie and Dorothy are here, Marsh. They wanted to be here with us."

That was fine. Millie and Dorothy were among my special friends from work. They were both Mother's age, but each had become my personal friend. Each was a special influence on my life. I was glad that they were here for Barbara and Pat.

Where is Dr. Kennedy? Why is this taking so long? Just as I thought about Dr. Kennedy, another doctor came into the emergency suite.

"Marsha, I'm Dr. Gonzales. Dr. Kennedy has been called out on another emergency. I am his associate. I will be taking care of you tonight."

I was disappointed.

"Couldn't another doctor take the other case?"

"I know, Marsha. It's so much better when your own doctor can be here, but he'll be in the first thing in the morning. I'll also call him tonight."

"But, Dr. Gonzales, you don't know my case." I began to feel trapped. Boxed in. In prison. Why didn't my opinion count? It seemed that when one of the physicians or other medical personnel wanted to know something, he or she would ask Barbara. I could barely overhear the staff in the hall discussing my unusual case. I stretched my head to hear.

"Hey, over here. The one on the bed. Ask me what's going on. I am very familiar with *my* history."

I laid in the emergency intensive care unit what seemed like forever. At least five different doctors came in to get the facts.

"Why don't we record this? That way you will have a permanent record of what has happened," I said.

Everyone seemed to be acting a little strange, I felt. But I tried to remind myself that I had never before nearly died. Maybe this was normal behavior. Over and over, I told them my history:

> I got sick last summer. I lost weight. The hospital felt it was a virus from the trip I had just taken or maybe even related to systemic sarcoidosis. I got better but continued to lose weight. I began to see Dr. Kennedy in the fall. He followed up with Dr. Johnson. I have already had nearly every test offered at this hospital. At this point, Drs. Kennedy and Johnson have evidence of the malabsorption syndrome. They still do not know why I have this. I also have an autonomic-something syndrome which causes the unpredictable heartbeats and the extremely low blood pressure. I have had rheumatic fever, pneumonia three times, the chicken pox, and a broken wrist, foot, finger, and toe. I have never had my tonsils or my appendix out. I still have not had the measles or mumps. I am not allergic to any drugs, and I have insurance.

"Sounds like you've had to go through this before."

I continued to wait. I stretched my head again to see if I could determine what they were going to do with me next. I could tell that there was a meeting in the hall right outside the trauma treatment room. I overheard words that I had heard before: *anorexia nervosa*. By now, I knew what they meant. They thought my weight loss was intentional. I wanted to defend myself, but I could not. After all, they did not know me. I was not their patient. Dr. Kennedy was not there to set them straight. I was mortified. The feelings became intense. I wanted to escape. I felt I was being accused. But what else could they think? After all, I did fit the profile. I was a dehydrated and emaciated woman.

Barbara comforted me. "No! You can't let that matter. Don't be intimidated by them, Marsh! They are simply doing their jobs. Besides, soon Drs. Kennedy and Johnson will be able to show them the records and charts. Now, relax."

Barbara was right. It should not have mattered, but it did. I tried to convince myself that I did not care what they thought, but I knew deeply that I did care. I felt I was being accused of trying to commit a sophisticated form of suicide. Hours earlier, I was fighting for my life. Now they are saying I caused this near-death experience.

I felt I was entering my own prison. But I had no keys to escape. No one had ever given me keys that unlocked such prisons of accusation. I felt the cold wind of winter again rushing in. The icy accusation was intense and piercing. I was not emotionally or spiritually armored for such a winter. I was unaware of any possessions I had to protect myself from this storm.

Reflections on Judgment

I never knew that I held the only set of keys available to unlock my own prison door of how I judged myself. Letting another person's perception of who I was became more important than my own, that gives the keys to others and slams the prison door in my face.

Unfortunately, your perception of yourself, as well as mine, has been more shaped from the outside in than the inside out. Other people tell us all of our lives who we are, what to do, and how to feel. Eventually, we believe that in order to be loved and accepted, we must be these things. This sets in motion the cycle of trying to live up to others' expectations. We become prisoners of what other people believe.

I do not have to be a victim of other people's assumptions. Instead, I can be transformed by the pain of accusation.

Part II
The Winter
A Time to Weep

An Anatomy of Pain
Solo Flight
Afraid of the Dark

I was born of pain
It is the clarifier of all our lives
Why do we fear it so?
For to live without pain is not to live.

But the vicious dragon
Wounds my body and now my soul
My pain is only lessened
As hot coals of deeper anguish penetrate to the bone.

Where can I run from this desperation
That sabotaged my life and breath
Nowhere can I go that pain does not meet me there.
But wait! Where can I go from Your Spirit?

The days are long,
The nights a mirage of desperate confusion
My soul is tossed in the winds of delirious debris.
This black dross that burns through the night
Can it burn within my spirit a new awakening?

Slowly, I hear You whisper
Be still . . . know that I am who I AM
Dear child, My love suffers long
Look at My hands, scarred and torn apart.
My pain has made you free
My love suffers long.

Oh, Father! Can my pain warm my soul?
Will it bring me gain, joy, and good?
Is this Your way to make pure gold?

Yes, You too were born of suffering
Only You know what I feel.

So, warm my soul with the coals that can purify
Carry me through another night
Awaken in me Your enduring heart
A wild and tenacious vision of life
And a heart more tender
Fused by the fire
Pure gold.

—MARSHA SPRADLIN

4
An Anatomy of Pain

For a little while you may have had to suffer grief
in all kinds of trials.
These have come so that your faith—
of greater worth than gold,
which persishes even though refined by fire—
may be proven genuine and may result in praise,
glory and honor when Jesus Christ is revealed
(1 Pet. 1:6*b*-7).

March 1984

Darkness filled the room even though it was still day. The clock's hands moved slowly, but moments were passing. I was still locked in the emergency ICU, waiting to be released to a room. Barbara came in frequently to cheer me on.

"I called your mother."

"Barbara, please, quick, tell her not to come."

"I knew you wouldn't want that, Marsha, but I had to. I called her from the condo while we waited for the paramedics. It was something I had to do for *me*."

"When will she arrive?"

"Millie and Dorothy are leaving shortly to meet her plane. She got a commuter flight out of Mobile but had to be routed through Houston because of bad weather. Come on, Marsha. Let us in."

I was experiencing mixed feelings. I wanted her to be with me, but I did not want her to come. Her arrival would be a public announcement that ol' Marsh had finally given in. My body was so weak, but my pride was still strong and more stubborn than ever.

Barbara squeezed my hand. "Love ya, kid! I'll be back in a minute."

By late that evening, my condition had stabilized enough for me to be released to a room. Before I was moved, someone shoved a pen into my hand. "Sign these, please, Miss Spradlin. They are just the regular papers saying we are not responsible for anything."

As I signed, I thought, *Who is responsible? Somebody must assume responsibility. That's a fact of life. If I was not guilty, then who was? Someone must take the blame.*

As the bars on the bed were pushed upward and locked into place, I felt the bars on my life locking me in. These were new sensations for me. I was unable to explain what I felt or why.

Attendants once again clustered the IVs together with the monitors. Two young men and a female nurse then strolled me through the maze of hallways of shiny glasslike floors. The lights on the ceiling flashed as we moved swiftly down the halls. Before getting too far, they stopped suddenly, and I saw Millie and Dorothy. I never knew how good it could be to recognize two sweet friends. They said absolutely nothing. They couldn't. I joked, I am sure.

"Must go, Miss Spradlin. She's going to be in room 6435. It's an end room, I believe. In fact, it is one of the four rooms here with two windows. Millie and Dorothy both leaned over and kissed my cheek. "Gone to get your mom!"

Barbara and Pat caught up. Pat smiled as we rolled onto the elevator. "Marsha, who called the hospital administration? You must have connections around here. You have a great room."

"What's the big deal about the room? I'm not planning on spending the week, just the night. Mother will be sorry she came."

"Sixth floor! Everybody off." The little caravan of my friends and hospital employees shuffled to the end of the hallway. Everybody was carrying something. Barbara had my tennis shoes. One nurse was pushing three poles with IV bags hanging off them. Two were pushing me. Another was in charge of the monitors.

"It's that end room. Careful! Swing her around carefully."

Getting the patient-transport bed inside the door was a real trick. I wanted to jump off and walk in. I felt ridiculous letting everyone make over me like I was an invalid. "Let me just walk into the room."

"Absolutely no way. Hospital policy!"

Oh well! It is easier to get forgiveness than special permission here, too, I thought.

"Marsha, pretend you're on vacation. Relax!" Pat was trying hard to help me settle down.

"Pat, this may be fun for some folks, but with all the creativity I have ever exhibited, there is no way I can compare this to a vacation. But I will say, the room is nice!"

"Look at this wallpaper. Can you believe it? It matches your bathroom."

It was exactly the same. A beautiful blue-and-beige stripe— my favorite colors.

Everyone helped move me to the bed. Once settled, I received the regular speech on how to make the bed go up and down, turn on the TV, and even control the curtains. I thought, *If I were not so sick, I could certainly enjoy this.*

"If you need anything, simply push this button. We will be in and out all night. Try to rest."

Barbara and Pat stayed for a few minutes, making sure I was settled and stable, both emotionally and physically. They agreed to go home and try to sleep. My ordeal had come the day before a major meeting of the executive board of our organization. All five of us—Barbara, Pat, Dorothy, Millie, and I—had major responsibilities. "I guess I'll miss the board meeting," I said.

"You'll be missed. But, Marsha, look at it this way. What better time for this to happen? Tomorrow, some of the greatest pray-ers in this state will be here—in this city. They all know you and love you. The timing is perfect. So, rest. I don't mean sleep. I mean *rest* in the Lord. He is here. When I think about all the things that happened today—the timing, the door being unlocked, my surprise visit, Pat's visit, the expert medical team —I am overwhelmed at the way the Lord has taken care of you. I don't understand all of this, Marsh, but I had such a peace. I knew what to do. Let's rest."

Barbara was a spiritual warrior. She was a friend but also a model of one who lived a life that reflected His love and compassion. I loved her, and I felt loved.

After Barb and Pat left, I was alone for the first time since lunch. My mind reminded me of a tape player racing forward and backward trying to find a certain piece of information. I could not grasp all that had happened. I seemed to either have no feelings, or my feelings were too explosive to handle. Although I was no longer in a physical state of shock, my emotions were. I felt that the Father had put a cushion inside of me to protect my emotions from the total impact of the day's experiences. I needed the energy simply to hang on. But, bit by bit, the impact was starting to seep in.

I had been sedated, but I did not sleep that night. At some point, a nurse came in with juice and drugs and caught me crying. She was a Hispanic woman about forty. She sat on the side of my bed, took my hand, and said, "Your mother called. She's in Dallas; I think she'll be here soon. I looked at your chart. You've had a rough day. Do you want to talk?"

I thought I was fine until I sensed her sympathy. Then tears flooded. I felt a need to explain. "I'm not anorexic. I didn't do this to myself. Do you believe me?"

"Honey, it doesn't manner. No one here cares about that. We just care about you. But if it'll make you feel better, I believe you. Besides, Dr. Kennedy will be here tomorrow. He will clear that up. Right now, I want you to take these. I think you'll rest better. I'll leave this juice. You need to drink!"

Shortly after she left the door opened again. I was expecting

Mother, but I had no idea how glad I would be to see her. The moment she walked into the door, I felt safe and secure. What a relief. The childhood feeling of "now that Mother was here, everything would be all right" seemed to elevate my gloomy spirit. I felt hope slipping in.

Dorothy and Millie had shared the details with her and assured her that I was critical but considered stable. I knew explanations were not needed for Mother. She did not need comforting, for she was a comforter by nature.

By the time she arrived, my condition had been upgraded from critical to guarded/stable, but Mother showed no real feelings. She had come prepared to fight. She was not going to let her emotions go up and down with every changing report. She was a warrior—one who could demonstrate enormous peace in the middle of a storm. She had total assurance that I was in the best of care. She chose to translate her negative energy of fear into positive energy of encouragement.

There was nothing anyone could say to convince Mother to go to my condo and sleep. She had come to be with me. She told Dorothy and Millie good-bye and then opened the closet and chest of drawers to unpack. "What are you doing? I'm the patient. Are you checking in, too?"

"Absolutely! If my girl is staying here, so am I. We're in this together for the duration. It's me and you kid. Let's just pretend we're college roommates! I'm sure there will be enough tests!"

"And where do you plan to sleep?"

"Scoot over!"

Mother crawled into my bed and simply held me. We cried, talked, prayed, and read the Bible, until nearly sunrise.

Dr. Kennedy breezed into my room around 7:30 AM. "You certainly pulled a good one. Last week I should never have let you talk me out of admitting you. Do you know what happened yesterday?"

I felt that Dr. Kennedy was *angry* at me. I had no idea he was actually *embarrassed*. He had promised Mother he would admit me days ago. He was right about one point: I had talked him out of it.

"What's the game plan, coach? When can I go home?"

"Go home! I just got you here, and all you can think about is going home! Marsha, my major concern right now is getting your weight up. It's dangerously low. I'm calling in a couple of doctors to consult today. I feel we may postpone all testing until we can get you up to at least ninety pounds. Let's see. Your weight today is eighty-two. That's two more pounds down this week. There has to be something we are missing."

The day lingered on. Nothing happened except that a computer mix-up meant that the cafeteria was sending me absolutely nothing to eat. By midday, I was starving.

Shortly after lunch, my room was filled with men in white jackets. Dr. Kennedy took the lead in explaining what needed to be done. The other doctors took notes and made suggestions. They were concerned that if I dropped another pound or two, I would go into another cardiac attack. They agreed that I should be placed on a form of life support. A device would be implanted through my neck into my heart to pump in a nutrient. This surgery would mean going to ICU. Mother and I agreed that I would do whatever was needed—but as we waited, nothing happened.

The day lingered on. We had no word from any of the physicians. Time was broken up with phone calls and the arrival of a dozen roses from the executive board of the organization I worked for. Mother remained calm, but I sensed that her patience was wearing thin.

A little after 4:00 PM, Dr. Kennedy plunged into the room. "Marsha, we have decided to abort surgery. We have your lab work. You're not manufacturing white blood cells. You count is about 3.0. That's very low. The risk of heart failure is also a critical concern, plus the idea of infection. There are simply too many risks. But we'll lose you if we don't turn this thing around . . . quick. At any moment, your heart could stop beating. We have decided to insert a tube into a section of your intestines. It will bypass the stomach. We already know your stomach is not absorbing nutrients, so we won't even try to go that route. You won't need to be in ICU, nor will we have to put you to sleep, even though it is a surgical procedure. That's not to say this is going to be pleasant, but you're a survivor. The surgeons will come for you shortly. Meanwhile, rest."

Mother walked into the hall with him. I am sure she pulled out additional information. I felt I understood and knew what I was up against. I knew what had to be done and felt like I had participated in the decision, but I felt that the conversation that had just taken place was about someone else. I felt fragmented and totally unattached to the pain.

The procedure went fine. Within an hour, I was back in my room. Five or six more plants arrived and stacks of cards. Word was out. I was very ill. I had mixed feelings about the attention, but it felt good to know so many people cared. I struggled with feelings of self-protection. As those first days turned into a week, I found myself withdrawing even more. I could not explain it. I did not want to see anyone. I felt guilt about the pain that Mother and Barbara were experiencing, but I also felt angry that it was happening to me. Dr. Kennedy was concerned about the depression. He was convinced I needed to be isolated from calls and visitors. My white blood count had now dropped to 2.6, and my weight was heading downward.

Each night, Mother and I would talk, cry, and read the "fan mail." Then I would get settled for bed while she called Daddy, Teresa, and Larry. I enjoyed hearing Mother and Daddy talk. They sounded like a couple of high school kids in love. She wrote him. He wrote her. Daddy cherished her letters. He saved each one.

Hi, Honey,

Do you miss me? Miss you, but glad I could come out. I think my being here has made it a little easier for Marsha. With Barbara tied up in an executive board meeting, it would have been rough.

We have a "no visitors" sign. Marsha gets real upset when anyone comes and stays over five minutes. The mornings are a little better, but she starts getting real depressed about four o'clock. She is just going through a bad time. I wish everyone could come out, but I am afraid she would be so depressed that it would hurt everyone more than not coming. She does not want to talk to anyone but Barbara. The problem is she thinks she has to be up for everyone, and she can't stay up.

She is also very self-conscious. She should be. You should see her, honey. Barbara and I just make her talk and cry out all the fears and feelings. That seems to be the only thing that helps. I just hope everyone can accept it for now and not feel rejected.

I have no idea when we will get her home. They took her off the IV yesterday to run more tests. She is back on IVs today. Her blood pressure is 70/40. Yesterday, she ate 4,600 calories and lost one more pound. But that really takes some of the pressure off. It tells the doctors the weight loss is not due to diet. She eats everything in sight.

I am doing fine. Barbara brought up an ice chest and all kinds of snacks. I will call if there is anything to report. Teresa and Larry are both calling. Why don't you three take turns? We must trust, Honey.

Love,

YOUR NUMBER ONE WIFE

I began to get even weaker. My emotions were shot. Sitting up in bed for more than ten minutes totally wore me out. I slept constantly. The days began to be fragmented. I felt as if I was losing the battle again. There was not one inch of my body that had not been stuck, poked, X-rayed, or listened to. Mother and I counted. In one day, eight doctors ran in and out of the room, each doing something to me. When all the other medical people were added, we had no room for me! Each physician seemed to have his own agenda, and each had his own set of questions. I was exhausted from going over the ordeal again and again. None of them gave a clue; none seemed encouraged. They each insisted, "When in doubt, order more tests."

Each morning, a nurse weighed me before anything else was done. And each morning, I weighed less. To ensure accuracy, the same nurse would roll the same set of upright scales into room 6435.

On the eighth day, I woke up disoriented. The ritual with the scales revealed that my weight had dropped sharply, overnight, to a stunning seventy-seven pounds. No way, not on 6,000 calories. I was terrified. I was losing. I was not in control. Nothing I did seemed to help. No amount of cooperation made things different.

Within moments, Dr. Kennedy and several lab technicians invaded my room with needles and procedures. Dr. Kennedy said nothing, but it was obvious that he was terrified, too. The blood tests were immediately sent to the lab. Dr. Gonzales came in minutes later with the results. This time he spoke to Mother, not me.

"Mrs. Spradlin, we are putting Marsha in ICU as soon as we can locate a bed. If this weight drops another ounce, I am afraid we will lose the battle. Her blood count is now in the lower twos and dropping. She must be quarantined."

"What's her blood pressure?"

Dr. Gonzales flipped through the pages of charts and records. When he spotted the blood pressure, he slammed the chart shut.

"No way!"

He took my arm and pumped the cuff: 60/40 and dropping. There was no time to spare. "Bed or no bed, we're moving you out of here!"

Later, we learned that my blood pressure readings were not accurate because of my lack of body fat. My blood pressure was much lower than any of the records showed. I should have been monitored with a "kiddie cuff"—not an adult cuff. This meant I should have been in ICU days ago.

Mother made two phone calls—one to Daddy and one to get a message to Barbara. Within minutes, a bed was available in ICU.

Attendants once again stacked blankets across my body. A rush of cold air swept over me. Then I felt the winter storm once again moving in. I shivered with the chill. The feeling was familiar. I was dying again!

They placed my fragile body on the transport bed, and the men in white jackets pushed me quickly down the congested hallways.

"Please, move to the side, please. We must move fast."

The lights began to flash again over my head as we rushed through the maze of hallways. My vision was blurred. Then, I saw red lights flashing. We had arrived. The lights meant there was an emergency. It was *me*. As I was pushed through the doors, I felt I was pushed into the storm—all alone this time. But those outside the door were encouraging me.

"Hold on tight."

I did. I wrapped my arms around my bony shoulders and held on tightly to my body. I was so afraid that the stormy winds would blow me off course.

Reflections on Pain

I've always wanted a life without pain. I viewed pain as something bad, evil, and undesirable. I did not realize that life without pain was impossible. Pain is as much a part of the human experience as joy. If viewed properly, pain can actually enhance life and joy.

Why, then, was I so afraid to hurt? I grew up thinking life was magic. My world was relatively pain free. Parents and teachers who go to great lengths to keep children from experiencing pain are doing them a disservice. Many children become adults, as I did, without going through a basic course in life's painful realities.

What are some positive side effects of pain? It can be our greatest teacher. It usually captures our total attention. Just as physical pain alerts us to the fact that something is wrong in our bodies and needs attention, emotional pain alerts us that there is a malfunction within our feelings. Immediate attention is required. If left untreated, like a mysterious or undiagnosed disease, it, too, will spread.

As I learned to listen to my pain, I learned something magnificent about myself. Likewise, I learned of the magnificence of the Holy Father. Regardless of its intensity or source, all pain—emotional, physical, or even spiritual—can be converted into an indispensable stimulus for positive change. But in order for that to happen, I must be willing to substitute something else for the pain. This may mean changing or shifting my perspective.

It seems that almost all of my emotional pain came through comparison. For example, I compared the way I felt to the way I once felt as well as the way I hoped to feel one day. I compared the way I looked to the way I used to look or hoped to look.

To relieve the pain, I had simply to be willing to give up the comparisons. That did not mean I ignored the pain or denied its existence. That would create more pain. Instead, I recognized it for what it was and what it was not.

Through my pilgrimage of pain, I learned that most of my emotional pain was self-made. It did not come from others, not even Jeff. That meant: No one was doing it to me. In most cases, I was doing it to myself. I was responsible for my emotional pain.

I began to realize that agonizing over my condition and trying to find someone to blame only intensified the hurt. This was an escape. I could choose to accept it and do something constructive with the negative energy it manufactured. Or, I could choose to agonize, resulting in more pain. The choice was mine.

With each action to reverse the negative energy, the pain decreased. Eventually, this became my only form of effective pain relief. It became addictive. I spent months in depression, feeling totally deprived of life, before I caught on to riding on the positive side of the wind.

This reminds me of the rose bushes in front of the house where I grew up. Each year Daddy would prune them so severely that they appeared ugly and nearly dead. But he knew what he was doing. I did not. He knew that pruning removed those parts of the bushes that were not needed, those parts that were a drain or burden on the rest of the plants. By removing them, the nutrients could go to the good plant parts, making the plants stronger and more beautiful. So it is with pain. I had to get rid of what I did not want to make room for what I did want. I realized that pain could either cut me, or it could serve me. It could trim me down, but not cut me down, unless I gave it full permission to do so. My survival instinct was far too strong to allow that.

I learned to view pain and joy as a part of the whole. They are interrelated and sometimes dependent and growing on each other. I realized that my continuous growth often depended on some discomfort. The amount of change I was willing to accept was in direct proportion to the amount of pain I was willing to experience.

I still reject pain. It still hurts, but I know I am not alone in pain. Jesus, too, has already experienced my every hurt. Oh, I wish I had known that during the winter of my pain!

Now, when tears come stealing my sight, and that still happens often, I dare to remember that He brought wisdom wrapped in pain. In the end, it is a gift.

What then is a proper response to pain? Rejoice!

Consider it pure joy, my brothers, whenever you face trials of many kinds, because you know that the testing of your faith develops perseverance. Perseverance must finish its work so that you may be mature and complete, not lacking anything (Jas. 1:2-4).

I still love the light, but I know that the road is sometimes darkest at the center line. It is there, hiding in deep shadows, that more lessons can be learned. I feel no need to drop bread crumbs behind as I travel the road by night. For me, His light shines brightest in the darkness of my stormy winter nights. His light can shine in your darkness, too.

All alone in the dungeon of my own deception and despair
I lie awake for hours wondering
When the candle will burn below the danger line
How long will my cradle swing over my own grave.

I know many are waiting in the wings
Remembering me
Loving me
Encouraging me to not give up hope.

Be a valiant warrior, they say
So with my sword and armor in place
I am destined to finish the race.

But if millions are cheering me on
Why do I feel I am fighting alone?
My only companion are the obstacles chilling the way.

With Your holy power as captain of my plight
I will be fearless and true
I will sing of my Redeemer
I will carry Your torch onward
I will carry it home.

Yes, I will sing of my Redeemer
For all alone, You purchased me
You sealed my pardon
You paid my debt
You set me free
All You ask of me is to keep up the fight.

I will carry His torch onward
But never alone
For You are the Valiant Courier
Bearing the flame that lights my way.

Together, we will run faster and harder
In this desperate relay
And to the end, we will carry the light
Until there is no more day.

—MARSHA SPRADLIN

5
Solo Flight

Consider it pure joy, my brothers,
whenever you face trials of many kinds,
because you know that the testing of your faith develops perseverance.
Perseverance must finish its work
so that you may be mature and complete,
not lacking anything
(Jas. 1:2-4).

March 17-28, 1984

Behind the red flashing light was my dark, sterile compartment in ICU. It was a dungeon. My cell was next to the wall. There were others in this sophisticated prison. Instead of bars, green curtains separated us. The machinery and gadgets accented the depression and darkness. But, as I was gently placed on the bed, I noticed a small window. It was shut tight and too far to reach, but it was a symbol of hope and a bond with the real world.

The physical pain had increased. But unlike the other three people in this neurological unit, I was awake. They were each on morphine or some other strong sedative. To relieve the pain, I was given Tylenol. The doctors believed that any stronger drug or chemical could trigger more weight loss. So, I was locked inside my own body. My only companion was pain. I had no way to escape. Regardless of where I was, the pain was there. But in ICU, it intensified.

Within the first hour, I became the focus of attention of the nursing staff. I needed attention, but I did not need the kind of attention I was getting. Nurses were adjusting the gadgets and machinery attached to every part of my body. I wanted warmth and comfort. I did not realize that ICU nurses are not used to their patients being awake. I wanted to be drugged. The sounds were intense. Clicks, alarms, beeps—each was amplified by the sound of the respirator breathing for the man whose bed was only inches from mine. He had been there for months. Learning that was no comfort to me.

Next to him was a young woman a little younger than I. She was totally unconscious. She had had brain surgery and was simply recovering. She was supposed to be placed in a room within a few hours.

Next to the other wall was the fourth patient—another woman about Mother's age, I guess. I learned less about her. She was there only two nights. She died. I watched it all. I heard the sounds. I wondered if that was what took place with me only days earlier. I wanted to help her, but I, too, was a victim waiting to be either sentenced or released. None of us held the keys to our prison cells.

It did not take long to memorize the tiny compartment. The green curtains were on one side, a green wall on the right. A gigantic clock was directly in front of me. Under the clock was a sink. At the foot of my bed was a computer. The staff told the computer every move I made. It became an extension of myself. Everything was documented. Instead of using the telephone to call for help, the nurses simply told the computer. They used it to order my Tylenol as well as to check my vital functions. It was hospital efficiency par excellence. As physicians came to check my status, they seldom spoke to me. Instead, they communicated with the computer. Information stations were located around the hospital. This made it easy for doctors to get updates on their patients. I wondered what the computer knew that I did not. Maybe it held the secret to my release.

The lights were on twenty-four hours straight. The nurses worked eight-hour shifts. After only one day, I lost track of day and night. I could not see out the window. It was too high. I had a desperate need to know if it was daytime.

I never slept, or at least I was not aware of it. The day was fragmented by three visiting periods: one at 10:15 AM, one at 2:45 PM, and one at 7:15 PM. Visitors were limited to immediate family members only. My immediate family was increasing. Dad could no longer be held in Mobile. He drove all night to be with Mother and Barbara. Teresa and my brother-in-law Milt, as well as our brother Larry and his wife Cindi, followed Dad one day later. They arrived late during my second night in ICU. I remembered hearing my brother outside the double doors trying to come in. He had driven for twelve hours and insisted on seeing me. The nurses stood their ground and denied his request. He was explosively angry. I could hear him crying and begging the staff: "I just want to see her one minute. I won't upset her. Please, I have driven all night to get here in time." Regardless of his plea, he was denied permission. More and more, I felt like I was a prisoner. I had no control. I could not choose who to see or when to see them. The emotional pain was far greater than the physical pain at this point. I was in serious but "guarded" condition.

There were seven people who waited. The support from Daddy and other family members was good for Mother and Barbara. Barbara, of course, was included as family. Their presence communicated to me the seriousness of my condition. Each waited for a moment to be with me. Hotellike rooms were available in the hospital for families. Mine stayed in the ICU waiting room nearly all day, but they did have a place where they could lie down and get away from the tension of the waiting room from time to time.

Family members and I made the best of each visit. Mother brought me a notebook and pen, and we began to write messages to each other. Because the twenty-minute visits always passed so quickly, the messages seemed to bridge the time between them and help us feel together when we were apart. They also gave us something tangible to hold in our hands between times together. Writing gave me something to think about when I couldn't have contact with the outside world. Once in a while, a nurse would even take a message out to my family. And, occasionally, I was surprised to receive a message from them. Messages became a symbol of holding on—together.

March 19, 1984

Dear Mother and Daddy,
It's 5:00 AM. I've just had the best experience with Denise, my nurse. She explained why I was in ICU. Something about the heart rate was dangerously low because of the lack of fluids. I guess that is why I am on twice the amount of IV as I was when I entered the hospital. She said I was worse, but there seemed to be no explanation. Denise also told me what happened in the condo. When I lost consciousness, it was due to the lack of blood flow to the heart. This caused cardiac arrest. I remember that I thought I had died. Since then I have improved some, but for some reason I have started to dehydrate again. This is the number-one concern right now. The second concern is, of course, getting the weight stabilized. It seems to be a circle. I feel I am going through a revolving door. All exits enter more pain and the unknown. Why does Denise feel I need to know how serious it is?
Whatever, I think I have accepted it. "To God be the glory." Right? I know it will be a long road back. But the journey could give me plenty of time to get reacquainted with my Father and with each of you.
I am so glad Larry and Teresa are here. I feel I am ready to share the struggle. Now, let's all hang in there knowing that this, too, can teach us faithfulness. I am glad you are here. I love you!
Mom, I need some socks!
Ouch! Just got two more shots, two tubes of blood, veins are collapsing.
Love,
MARSHA

For no obvious reason, on the evening of March 18, my condition sharply declined. I only remember the nurses standing over me all night and tapping frantically on the keys of the computer. My heart rate dropped dangerously low to 28 beats per minute. My blood pressure barely existed. The reason for my survival was not obvious. But on March 19, the ICU waiting room began to be flooded with calls from friends and acquaintances across the United States who testified about being awakened in the middle of the night for no reason except to get out of bed and pray for "our Marsh."

On March 25, Mother slipped in first for the morning visit.

"Here, honey, sign this. It's a card for Barbara. Today is her birthday."

"Oh, Mother, I forgot. I can't remember. I didn't know it was daylight outside, and I don't even have a gift."

I panicked! Tears would not stop.

Mother broke down and cried freely in my presence for the first time. Our tears smeared the ink on the card.

When Barbara came in moments later, I pushed the card into her hand and continued to cry. "Oh, Barbara, I'm sorry. This' not such a great birthday for you. It's a nightmare. I need to give you something. Here."

I had on my right hand a little ring engraved with the symbols for the four seasons. It was among my most special possessions. I had managed to get into ICU with it on. I pulled it off and slipped it onto her little finger.

"No, Marsha. I can't take your ring. You love that ring. I'm just glad you're still alive. That's the best gift I could possibly get."

Barbara soon realized that not taking my ring would be far more disappointing to me. She accepted reluctantly but graciously.

I grieved all day. I felt I was entering another level of deep depression. I no longer cared if I lived or died. I only wanted to be with my friend on this day. Instead, I was having my own party—a pity party. I was tired of trying, fighting, and caring.

By noon, one of my doctors came in with my parents.

"Marsha, we feel we must take a more careful look at the possibility of leukemia. Your white blood count is looking more like leukemia every day. The evidence is mounting.

"Your body simply isn't reproducing white blood cells. They are necessary to fight infections, not to mention to live. I have ordered a spinal tap and a bone marrow test. We must look into the possibilities. You won't be put to sleep, but it won't be pleasant. I just wanted you to know what we're telling your parents and what we're up against. Now rest!"

Sure! Just like that—rest!

Within the hour, a young surgeon came into my little corner of the room. His hands were loaded down with green cellophane-wrapped packages of surgical supplies and all kinds of liquid solutions.

"Roll to your side."

"Wait! Please, Dr. Carter. I want to be with her when you do it," Debbie, my favorite ICU nurse, insisted.

Dr. Carter waited while Debbie scrubbed. Debbie then moved to the left side of the bed and gently knelt, placing her hands on mine.

"Babe, what ya say we pull this one off together? You squeeze my hand. Pretend that the harder you squeeze, the more you're able to control and decrease the pain. All right. Ready, Dr. Carter?"

I held on tight. Dr. Carter and the others were right. The pain was intense. Suddenly, a sharp, striking pain split through my every fiber like a bolt of lightning, shocking my entire body, not leaving a nerve untouched.

I jerked suddenly toward Debbie.

"Oh, no, I'm so sorry, Marsha! The needle slipped off the spine. I know this must be incredible. I promise, this never happened to me before. I just never have tried to do one of these on somebody so small and with such brittle bones. I've got to try again. Marsha, come on, Dear, one more time. I promise not to mess up again. If I do, you can do this to me. OK?"

Debbie looked at Dr. Carter as if to say, *You jerk!*

'Tell ya what, Marsha, I have a surprise planned. When we finish this, let's have a picnic."

Debbie already had prepared compresses. They were instantly placed against my swelling back. I was so overcome with the sudden, intense pain that I had heard nothing anyone had said. I felt nauseated and faint.

"Hold on. One more time, and we're through."

In a weak, faint voice I pleaded, "Please, no. Don't do it anymore. Will you leave? I don't care if I have leukemia. I simply don't care."

The second attempt was successful. I was rearranged in my bed and given a shot for the pain. I was unable to move or even feel anything for hours. The accident was documented on the computer. It was already permanently on file in my mind and emotions. In many ways, it deepened my feeling of being sub-human. I felt Debbie was my only tangible symbol of hope, justice, and mercy.

My condition continued to worsen during the evening. Later, I learned that again I was a candidate for cardiac arrest. Months after the experience, Debbie shared with me the desperate and helpless feelings she, Denise, and the others had. She described the pain they experienced while watching the monitor and knowing there was no reason I should still be alive. Each heartbeat should have been the last. They knew that with each breath they were observing a miracle. My survival was not "supposed" to happen. But my heart evidently had not picked up the message to die. I was told I said to Denise during the night, "If you can't trust your own heart, what can you trust?"

Near the end of the first week in ICU, the team of eight

physicians met with Mother and Daddy and my immediate family to discuss their game plan. Dr. Kennedy's mother was ill, so he could not be there. Prior to the meeting, one physician came in to share with me the position of the staff. I could tell he had some heavy news. I did not know a rumor was stirring.

"Marsha, I believe in you, but I am a doctor. There are so many unanswered questions, and we need to know why: the white blood count, for one thing. The team of physicians believe you may have anorexia. I am not saying I believe that, nor do many of the other doctors. We are actually split right down the middle. The fact is, we have had our own wars over it. Some say maybe—others say absolutely not. The fact is, we are saying we are willing to investigate the possibility. You understand that, don't you? We can't leave a stone unturned. We must look at everything.

"Are you accusing me of trying to do this to myself?"

"Nobody is accusing you of anything. We are doctors. We are having to look at our own reputations."

"Wait, just because you can't seem to come up with a direct relationship between the weight loss and some known illness, you now assume that it's me?"

"Marsha, calm down. We simply must investigate this."

"Investigate!" I felt the anger building. "What exactly are you saying? How do you explain my losing five pounds since I entered the hospital on 6,000 calories a day?"

"Some women throw up."

"What? Because some women do it, then you're assuming I do it, too? I've been watched for days. When do I do this?"

"Marsha, I really must go now. Your parents are waiting."

As he left, my eyes stormed with tears and anger. Debbie had heard the whole thing. She came and embraced me.

"Marsha, you're innocent. I can't believe doctors. When they don't know what causes something, they assume it's in your head. Such pride. I know. I work with them all the time."

"Whatever happened to 'innocent until proven guilty?' "

Two hours passed. It was now time for the afternoon visit. I was eager for Mother and Daddy to come. I knew they would probably have a story about how they set the record straight with the doctors. They knew me.

Mother entered my corner compartment first. She was alone. Her eyes were bloodshot. She had been crying.

"Mother! What's wrong? Don't tell me . . ."

"Marsha, I'm going to ask you only this one time. Listen carefully, Honey. Are you doing this to yourself? Because if you are, you must know that you are killing us, too."

I could not speak. *My own mother now has lost faith in me,* I thought. Finally, with my voice quivering, I tried to tell her.

"Mother, don't you know me?"

Suddenly my hope was drained. As long as I had my family pulling for me, I felt I could hold on. Now I had nothing. I felt totally alone.

"Marsha, we are just terrified. The doctors do care about you, Honey. I know you don't think that. They all do. You have always had a charisma with people. They don't want to believe it; none of us do. We just have to know."

"No! I've never thrown up. It makes me sick to think about it. You know I eat. You've lived with me for weeks."

"Of course, Honey."

"Do you believe me?"

"OK, I just had to hear it from you. Your dad and I will fight for you. I know you feel you are in this thing alone. Come on, chin up! Barbara wants badly to see you. Try to dry those tears and be up for her."

In many ways, the war was on. Inside, I knew I was now on a solo flight. Would I ever trust anyone again? Would I ever feel that I was trusted? The next weeks were ones of proving.

A nurse was instructed to watch my every action. I was indeed a prisoner, captured and defeated, but innocent.

Again, communicating with the outside world was my only form of emotional maintenance. I wrote:

March 25 1984

Dear Family:

It's ten minutes until visiting hours again. I must apologize for being so down at the last visit. This must be real hard on you all, too! Maybe harder. I know some of your feelings. I must be strong for you. The Lord has given me a peace, I think, or at least I am expecting it to come real soon.

Debbie just left. She stopped and gave me a hug before leaving. We have really grown to love each other. I can talk to her. I trust her. I really love her. We spend hours just talking. I think she trusts me. Hey, she is a Catholic. She told me she prayed for me in mass.

I think I have figured out some of my depression. I was just having a selfish pity party. Please know that while you eat birthday cake, I am drinking, via tubes, 500 CCs of ISOTIS HP. Would you like to have a bottle to go with your birthday cake? It should cure all that ails you. How about your sending in some cake to go with my ISOTIS HP. I am glad my stomach is not having to digest this stuff. Yuk!

Pam, my night nurse, said I really was where I should be. Maybe there are other nurses that needed a witness. I don't think Pam is a Christian. She did tell me my records showed that for the first two nights I was once again a candidate for cardiac arrest. The lowest beat was in the upper twenties. I guess that is why I felt so sluggish. She said they can't put me on my regular heart drugs until the pulse gets up. I'm sort of on my own.

The good news is that my charts are indicating nearly 100 percent eating. This must be frustrating those doctors to death.

I am listening to the tapes Teresa and Milton left me. I am sorry they are all going to have to go back. But they had better get back to "my kids."

The notes and letters help. Please forgive me for my occasional depression. I just got so used to having Mother spoil me in room 6434.

I now know why this is called "guarded" condition.

We must keep trusting. Remember, "all things do work for
good for those that love Him."
Love,
MARSHA

I badly wanted and needed to get out of ICU. Debbie was
sensitive to my desire to get in touch with the outside world,
so she arranged to take me outside briefly on one of the private
patios. The sunshine's brightness stung my eyes. But its
warmth seemed to have a soothing affect. I had forgotten how
much I had missed the sun! Even though the experience was
medicine to my soul, my body was unable to adjust. I realized
how weak I had become. The sharp contrast between the outside brightness and the "dungeon's" darkness was depressing.

Debbie continued to find excuses to free me from ICU—
regardless of how brief the escape. I was granted permission to
be carried down the hall for a shower. Real hot water and
soap—I never thought I would ever be so excited about those
two things. Denise went with me. I had forgotten, in the excitement, that I was being watched. Denise helped untangle
the tubes and the other gadgets. Slowly the hospital gown
dropped to the floor. I stood there, totally naked. A mirror was
plastered all over the wall next to the shower. I was unable to
avoid seeing my reflection. I was horrified and emotionally
unprepared for what I saw.

My face was masked in white tape and bandages used to
keep the tubing in place and avoid infections. My neck, chest,
back, one hand, and one arm were all attached to other tubes.
Another hand and arm were in a splint devised to keep my
already collapsing veins from becoming even weaker. Six
monitoring devices were attached to my chest and side. My
hair was tangled, my skin cold and dry. My eyes were almost
shut. One was nearly closed entirely. I looked at Denise.

"I can't stay in here, Marsha. Don't tell a soul, but I'm going
to pull up a chair outside this door. You need privacy."

I turned the water on and slowly moved into the shower. The stinging hot water felt fantastic. The force of the shower weakened my disguised body. Slowly, I bent forward until my face touched the floor. I could not avoid the tears. The pouring water brought forth a steady stream of emotions, hidden feelings, and creepy fears. It was an internal cleansing as well as external. I cried and screamed.

"Dear God. Please, take this away. Please, make it be a dream. Make it be over. I feel so cold and so alone. It is the winter of all my years. Don't let this be true. I don't care if I die; I don't think I can stand living like this anymore. Please help!"

A sudden knock on the door startled me. "Are you all right in there?"

"Yea, just a minute."

There was something very therapeutic about the shower. I was *alone*! As the water streamed down my body, tears streamed down my face. It was a moment simply to say what I felt to the only One whom I was convinced really cared. I rested that night. For the first time in days, I had complete privacy.

The morning brought with it the usual routine. After the humiliating sponge bath, I was weighed—but not like a normal person. The staff wheeled in another machine that had a basket-type device attached. The basket was lowered, and my completely naked body was rolled into it. Then the basket was lifted, suspending me in midair. The machine measured my weight ounce by ounce and documented the information in the computer.

The emphasis on weight was intense. I began to resent people who complained about being a few pounds overweight. I would cherish having that problem.

I remained in ICU for over a week. Debbie became my advocate. She finally had the occasion to corner one of the physicians and simply describe what she had documented. In fact, she really risked her job. She was convinced of my innocence. She also insisted that regardless of my white blood count, I needed to get out of ICU. It was for people who were not awake, and emotionally, it was killing me. According to Debbie, the physician could not have agreed more.

"No one really believes she is anorexic except one doctor. And, he's the boss until Dr. Kennedy get's back. I'll do what I can, Debbie."

It worked. Later the next evening, Dr. Gonzales came in with the announcement.

"How would you like to get out of here, young lady? I heard about an opening up on the sixth floor. It's not your old room, but it's close. But before getting too excited, you have to play along with me. There are still those who are trying to convict you. Here's the plan. A private nurse will have to be assigned to you every moment until we get enough documentation to prove you are not anorexic."

"Then what? More tests?"

"Let's take this one day at a time. But remember, the nurse is not there just to watch. You can't be left alone. On a good day, your blood pressure is still low enough for shock. We really are in a better position to take care of you in here. Are you ready to risk leaving ICU?"

"Gladly! I'll accept this gift of freedom, but please, not a nurse. Why not Mother?"

"Marsha, I've outlined your options. It's a nurse or stay right here."

I was placed exactly where Dr. Gonzales said. The room was *not* my beautiful room with the two windows. It was a typical hospital room—dreary. I think Mother was as disappointed as I was.

I had been there only moments and settled on my egg-crate mattress (to lessen the pain of lack of body fat) when she walked in: a dumpy sergeant-type nurse. Her greeting was simple.

"Marsha, I'm Mrs. King. I already know that you don't want to see me, but you're stuck with me."

I spoke not a word.

As I sat up in bed to eat breakfast, she pulled out a notebook and a pen and began recording every move. Having to swallow with all kinds of tubes and gadgets either inside my throat or attached to it made eating difficult. But having "Sergeant" King watching and noting every bite of egg I put in my mouth made me even more nervous.

My anger built. I could not control it. I felt that I hated her. I knew I should not hate, but I was so lonely. Won't someone rescue me from this nightmare, wake me up, tell me it's a dream? There was no one to help relieve the pressure. I only wanted to reserve my emotions and strength to fight to live.

Perhaps it was the anger that made me want to test her. I got up from my bed, one of my first times to actually walk, and managed to pull the IV poles toward the bathroom. I started to close the door.

"Oh no, you don't! No tricks with me, young lady."

"Please! I just wanted to brush my teeth. Write that down in your notebook. Is there anything wrong with brushing your teeth?"

"Honey, I know this makes you mad. I don't like it either."

"Leave! Leave me alone. Get out. Please! Just leave!"

Daddy was standing in the hall and had overheard the conversation. He rushed into my room. His eyes revealed the sorrow he felt.

"Honey, what's wrong? Is there a problem?"

"Daddy, you've always been able to make things OK. Can't you make her go away? Why won't anyone trust me? Please, Daddy. You've always taken care of me. Please!"

Daddy's already bloodshot eyes began to flood with tears. "Baby, you know Daddy would. I can't! Not this time. We have got to trust the doctors."

Daddy held me to console me. But once again I felt abandoned. I was rejected. No one trusted me. My feelings did not seem to count anymore.

I lay there staring into space. My focus was on one corner of the wall. I must have stared into silence for one hour. My spirit was unable to cry. The moments were like momentum—thrusting time against me. The thrust was an intense emotional pain, unlike the physical pain I had known. It resembled the rushing wind just before a winter storm. The wind was cold and intense. I felt naked in the cold with nowhere to go, no shelter, no security, no love, no hope, all alone to make a solo flight into the rushing wind of the storm. *I will have to fly alone.* I was frightened since I had never flown that course before. What would I learn on my solo flight? Would I ever meet trust again? Would I ever know love? Would there ever be peace and acceptance? Quietly, I waited to take flight. Slowly, I put on an armor of protection to guard my emotions for the winter that was rushing in.

Reflections on Solitude

Life is a solo flight. We all experience it alone. From the moment we are born, we are in the world but detached from it. For many, life is lonely. To feel that no one has ever known our kind of pain or loneliness is absolute truth. No one has. No one can.

Feelings are personal. No one has access to your feelings. No one can feel what you do. Regardless of how much you desire to share them or move your burden to someone or something, it simply can't be done. And that brings up the value of accepting and learning to like solitude.

Solitude is that positive force that yields security and serenity. Where does it come from? It is a gift from the Good and Perfect Giver. Our Father gives us solitude. It comes by choosing to be alone with the only One who *does* know how we feel and the intensity of our pain.

Solitude, when do we feel it? Ah, it is the calm in the midst of the rushing winds of our own personal winters. It is the quietness and confidence we experience as growth and completeness become an antithesis of loneliness (Isa. 30:15).

Solitude, why do we need it? Silence causes great things to happen and be fashioned in our lives. During the quietness of solitude, we become one with ourselves and with God. We gain the momentum to fly into the storm, not be devastated by it. We gain the momentum to be ones who are leaned on rather than ones who always need to lean.

Solitude, what are the side effects? When we spend time with our Creator, we recognize Him in His magnificence. We likewise recognize our own magnificence. We learn of our gifts and our abilities. We accept ourselves as snowflakes—His unique creation for the winter. We learn to enjoy our uniqueness and gain insights on how we can contribute to the quality of life for others.

Solitude, where does it take place? Solitude calls our attention to the two worlds in which we live: The world and the way the world thinks; God's world and the way God thinks. In the solitude of His love, these two worlds are reconciled.

So why do we spend our lives trying to escape solitude? Because we have defined it as *loneliness.* Loneliness brings fear.

Fear of loneliness can only be conquered through solitude. When we discover solitude, we commune with the Only One who knows our pain. For nothing we experience did our Savior not likewise experience.

So, take your broken wings. Allow the Good and Perfect Giver to mend your wings for your solo flight above the storm.

Darkness has intruded my soul
Like an unwelcomed guest
Black clouds surround my spirit
Squeezing out my life
Blinding my sight.

I call to You, kind Father
I look for you in my despair
But I cannot hear Your voice
Nor can I see.

My dreams have turned into nightmares
Please! Call my name
Hear my cry, Oh Lord
My heart is overwhelmed
Lead me to the rock that is higher than I.

Quickly, just now
Awaken me
Chase the night's dark clouds away with Your holy light
Fill my eyes with Your visions of hope and joy.

Come soon
Let the morning light
Fill every corner of this gloom
Please!
Hear my cry, oh Lord
You are welcomed here.

As Your dawn conquers this darkest hour
Conquer my fear of the dark despair
Bring peace to still the quiver in my soul
Fill my life with the light that comes
Only at the end of blackest nights.

But, if I should die before I wake
Awaken me, gentle Father, as Your child
For then my soul shall know forever
The radiant glow of the eternal day.

—MARSHA SPRADLIN

6
Afraid of the Dark

You will not fear the terror of night,
nor the arrow that flies by day,
nor the pestilence that stalks in the darkness,
nor the plaque that destroys at midday
(Ps. 91:5-6).

Late March-April 1984

I lay very still in my bed. I was locked in mid emotion. These were days of confused situations and nights of restless remorse. My heart and soul lay wounded as a corpse.

I thought release from ICU would bring freedom from the prison. It would be a refuge. No, I could not escape the prison. I laid there listening. Surely I would hear someone dangling the keys. I had not yet learned that freedom is not a place; it is a state of mind. I was locked in the darkness of my own lack of openness to be taught by the One who held the keys.

I was still unable to say exactly what I was so desperately afraid of. If I were not anorexic, then I was real. If I were real, why did I feel such emotional pain? Questions about my fear continued to swim in my head. It was not physical warfare; it was spiritual. My life and emotions had become a spiritual battleground.

Slowly, I reached for my Bible. My eyes were dry. There were no tears left. My eyes scanned the pages of my old, well read brown-leather Bible. I read every marked passage that had spoken so much to me in earlier days of trial and pain. Nothing! Nothing unlocked the prison door of my fear. Then I ran across one book in which I had nothing marked—Lamentations. The

name described me. I felt a spark of hope. *Maybe Lamentations.*
There, I read a profile of myself from Lamentations 3:1-39,47-
50,54-58, and I changed the pronouns to make it personal:

I am the woman who has seen affliction
Because of the rod of His wrath.
He has driven me away and made me walk
In darkness and not in light.
Surely against me He has turned His hand
Repeatedly all the day.
He has caused my flesh and my skin to waste away,
He has broken my bones.
He has besieged and encompassed me with bitterness and hard-
ship.
In dark places He has made me dwell,
Like those who have long been dead.
He has walled me in so that I cannot go out;
He has made my chain heavy.
Even when I cry out and call for help,
He shuts out my prayer.
He has blocked my ways with hewn stone;
He has made my paths crooked.
He is to me like a bear lying in wait,
Like a lion in secret places.
He has turned aside my ways and torn me to pieces;
He has made me desolate.
He bent His bow
And set me as a target for the arrow.
He made the arrows of His quiver
To enter into my inward parts.
I have become a laughingstock to all my people,
Their mocking song all the day.
He has filled me with bitterness,
He has made me drunk with wormwood.
And He has broken my teeth with gravel;
He has made me cower in the dust.
And my soul has been rejected from peace;
I have forgotten happiness.

So I say, "My strength has perished,
And so has my hope from the Lord."

Remember my affliction and my wandering, the wormwood
and bitterness.
Surely my soul remembers
And is bowed down within me.
This I recall to my mind,
Therefore I have hope.
The Lord's lovingkindnesses indeed never cease,
For His compassions never fail.
They are new every morning;
Great is Thy faithfulness.
"The Lord is my portion," says my soul,
"Therefore I have hope in Him."
The Lord is good to those who wait for Him,
To the person who seeks Him.
It is good that she waits silently
For the salvation of the Lord.
It is good for a woman that she should bear
The yoke in her youth.
Let her sit alone and be silent
Since He has laid it on her.
Let her put her mouth in the dust,
Perhaps there is hope.
Let her give her cheek to the smiter;
Let her be filled with reproach.
For the Lord will not reject forever,
For if He causes grief,
Then He will have compassion
According to His abundant lovingkindness.
For He does not afflict willingly,
Or grieve the daughters of men.
To crush under His feet
All the prisoners of the land,
To deprive a woman of justice
In the presence of the Most High,
To defraud a woman in her lawsuit—

Of these things the Lord does not approve.
Who is there who speaks and it comes to pass,
Unless the Lord has commanded it?
Is it not from the mouth of the Most High
That both good and ill go forth? . . .
Panic and pitfall have befallen us,
Devastation and destruction;
My eyes run down with streams of water
Because of the destruction of the daughter of my people.
My eyes pour down unceasingly,
Without stopping,
Until the Lord looks down
And sees from heaven. . . .
Waters flowed over my head; . . .
I said, "I am cut off!"
I called on Thy name, O Lord,
Out of the lowest pit.
Thou hast heard my voice,
"Do not hide Thine ear from my prayer for relief,
From my cry for help."
Thou didst draw near when I called on Thee;
Thou didst say, "Do not fear!"
O Lord, Thou didst plead my soul's cause;
Thou hast redeemed my life (adapted from NASB).

I read those words over and over. I couldn't believe how
appropriate they were for me. God does have a heart that tears
can touch. Like Jeremiah, I had been captured. There is no
valley so low that He is not there. If He could deliver Jeremiah
from his sorrows of Zion, surely He could likewise deliver me
and hear my prayer. Each time I read the verses, I realized
something of my own experience that exactly paralleled Jeremiah's. Here's my version:

I am a woman of affliction.
I have walked in darkness and not light.
I have felt that His hand has turned on me.
My flesh and skin surely wasted away.

I have become encompassed with bitterness.
I lived in the dark places of ICU.
I was walled in there.
I could not go out.
My chains of monitors and tubing wear heavy.
Even when I cry out for help, I feel shut out.
My way is blocked—"No visitors."
My path is crooked at the lack of solutions.
I feel I am being watched and ready to be devoured.
The arrows of Dr. Carter's needles have entered my most inward parts.
I feel I am the laughingstock of all people.
I feel mocked.
I am bitter.
I feel drunk with sedatives.
I feel as a cowerer in the dust.
My face is bent to the floor in search of help!
I feel rejected from peace and ripped from happiness.
I have no peace.
My strength has perished, and so has my hope from God.
But wait, God delivered Jeremiah.
I have hope.
The Lord's lovingkindnesses indeed never cease.
His compassions never fail.
They are new every morning;
I have hope!
Marsha, I am good to those who wait.
But wait silently for your salvation.
Sit alone—and seek Me.
I will not deprive you of justice.
Marsha, I know you have felt pain, devastation, and destruction.
I am aware that your eyes run down with streams of tears.
But now I am looking down at you from heaven.
I have heard your prayer for relief and your cry for help.
I am near.
Do not fear.

I will plead your case.
I will redeem your life.

I was freed. I knew that my devastation was not from God, but He allowed it. His allowing it simply implied His supreme authority over all things.

I was relieved to realize that my fear of death, my prison, was not from the mouth of the Most High. I examined my heart. I quickly returned to the Lord. I felt like I must lift up my heart and hands toward heaven. I was redeemed.

I made a covenant. I would wait. I would watch, and I would accept all—not just the good. But there was more. I would testify about all He had shown me. I had been afraid of death. No longer. I had peace with my Creator. As I released the fear of death, I learned that I was the one who had captured my own spirit and made myself a prisoner. Release from ICU was not a release from myself. Freedom is not a place. It is a state of mind and spirit—even with Sergeant King in my presence. I was freed. Before, there was no place I could go to get away from my prison; now there was nowhere I could go and not find freedom.

I began to feel energy for the first time in months. Where do I start? And when? I must prove that this freedom is real. My question was almost instantly answered. Dr. Gonzales walked in. An empty cereal bowl was on my tray. I had eaten its contents. Dr. Gonzales picked up the bowl and laughed.

"What kind of trick do you have planned for this?"

My Bible was still open. Sergeant King was sitting next to my bed, watching closely to see how I would react to Dr. Gonzales's accusation.

"Dr. Gonzales, I forgive you. It's OK that you feel that way. I know you are scared. I was, too. I did not know how much until now. I don't know if you are a Christian; I don't really know anything about you, but God just visited me. I know that sounds strange. But for the first time since I came here, almost three weeks ago, I am free. I am going to live. I am going to be able to tell about this. God will be praised. I really think something just happened. I feel good. I have been delivered. I want you to know that, Dr. Gonzales. I want you to know Him who just delivered me. I don't care what you say to me or what you do to me. I know I am OK."

I laughed for the first time in months.

Dr. Gonzales sat on my bed and said nothing but reached out and took my hand. He didn't examine my body; he was examining my soul. He didn't listen to the inconsistencies of my heart beating. He was listening to me. Or maybe it was Him that he was hearing.

Sergeant King became Mrs. King—my friend. She had seen a miracle—not physical but spiritual. By midafternoon, Drs. Gonzales and Johnson came in. Mrs. King greeted them.

"She doesn't need me anymore. She is OK."

"We know, Mrs. King. We have already decided to release you.

"And for you, young lady, you have just been pronounced 'not guilty.' How would you like to get that tube out of your throat? In fact, let's just do it right now, Dr. Johnson. How about letting her do it?"

"Why not?"

"Just pull it out. It doesn't hurt." Tears rolled down my checks. Happy ones. Slowly, I pulled on the tube.

"There is no end to this. Are you sure I will get to the end."

Drs. Gonzales and Johnson laughed. Mrs. King wiped her tears as she tried to hide her emotions.

"Why are you doing this, Dr. Johnson?" she asked.

"We don't know. I guess it has finally occurred to these stubborn doctors that, well, this is a Christian medical institution. If we can't trust the Great Physician, we are practicing the wrong kind of medicine. This is a miracle case. We already know that. Otherwise, you would not have made it this far. So,

why are we so afraid? I guess we, too, are terrified of death—
for anyone."

Mother and Daddy could not have timed it any better. They
walked into a party of happy friends celebrating life.

"More good news, honey. The hall supervisor just released
the patient in 6435. We can get back into our old room tomorrow morning."

It was a peaceful night; however, I did not sleep. I was not
used to darkness! Early the next morning, Mother convinced
Daddy to go home for a while. They owned a business that
demanded his attention. They agreed he would return to Dallas in a few days if needed. Before leaving, Daddy assisted in
moving me to "my" room. We unloaded plants and unpacked.
No one had asked how long we would be there. No one really
wanted to know. We were content, for now, to wait on the
Great Physician. He obviously was not finished.

Dad and Mom used two rolls of tape displaying the hundreds of get-well cards. Virtually every inch of wall space in
that large room was now covered. Hospital personnel from
every floor dropped by to see the display that had become the
talk of the hospital. Quite often, during routine tests, technicians read my name on one of my three arm bands and com-
mented, "Oh, you're the one with the cards. I heard about
them."

Saying good-bye to Daddy was one of the most difficult
moments I had at the medical center. I stood with Mother and
watched him walk across the lawn to the parking garage. I
noticed the grass was turning green. Life! Even in winter?

Daddy looked up and saw us standing at my window. Pain
filled my eyes. Mother and I did not say a word. We simply
held tightly to each other. Daddy and I both knew that I was
his little girl. Likewise, we knew the chances were still pronounced that he might never see his little girl again. Nothing
can explain that feeling. I have wondered how we were able
to do it. I had heard that "God doesn't give you dying grace

until you're dying." We had grace for every moment. As Daddy walked to the car, I wondered if I would ever walk to my car. I knew deeply that if ever I could do something so simple as walk to my car, I would forever be happy!

My condition did not improve. In fact, I began to show signs of decline. I heard rumors that I would be readmitted to ICU. It was OK this time.

"We can't sit back and do nothing. We are going to start from the beginning," announced Dr. Gonzales.

Doubts began to cloud my vision again. Like darts. I began to sincerely doubt if I would ever go home. Once again the testing began: countless X rays, CAT scans, body scans, electrocardiograms, pituitary tests, and volumes of blood tests. My last good vein finally collapsed. I wondered if my right hand would be permanently scarred. It was.

I was still listed in critical/guarded condition even though I was no longer in ICU. Visitors were still restricted; any germ could be the devastating blow. It was hard to enforce the rule, but we tried. Often people I did not even know would drop in to pray. Mother never left. While I did not know it, people were still expecting me to die. Dr. Gonzales had told Mother not to leave me. I could still simply stop breathing.

In the late evenings and early mornings, Barb came. Often she brought supper for Mother. We became a sort of sorority. I slept almost constantly during the day but lay awake during the night. I was still afraid of the darkness of the unknown. I was still afraid of dying. Often when I did fall asleep, I would awaken at 1:00 or 2:00 AM to find Mother standing over me. She would be touching my leg, arm, or have her hand on my head. She was afraid to sleep, thinking I might stop breathing. One of us was awake all of the time to make sure I was alive.

Once I awakened in the darkest part of the night to find that Mother wasn't there. I was terrified. Had I died? I screamed suddenly.

"Mother!"

She had stepped outside the room for a few minutes of fresh air. I had reacted like a three- or four-year-old child who is lost in a department store. Mother was apparently frightened by my voice. She ran into the room expecting the worse.

"I was just scared, Mother." I crawled into her lap—a thirty-year-old child. She held me all night, rocking me back and forth, calming me by stroking my brow.

What was I so afraid of? Dying! I simply didn't know how to die. I always wanted to do well in every endeavor. But I realized that no one had ever taught me how to say good-bye. My survival instinct was still strong, but I was beginning to realize that it, too, was once again slowly fading. I was afraid of being alone. Saying good-bye to those I loved seemed too painful to even think about. But saying good-bye to myself seemed impossible. How could I? I had never even known myself. How could I give away something I had not really had before? The darkness of the night represented the darkness of the unknown. I dreaded the darkness. I hated what I could not see. So, I struggled to remember Jeremiah and his lamentation. I tried to wait.

Reflections on Fear

Dying was my fear. We all have a survival instinct. We all probably believe that death is something that happens to someone else. But life for each of us is terminal. If we are not being born, then we are simply dying. How can we know and experience life fully if we are unable to accept the reality of our own mortality?

I felt that dying at such a young age would be devastating. Death was for older people, not me. I felt cheated. But soon I realized that time is relative. Many people can experience more life in a moment than others experience in a lifetime. But how much time is a lifetime? Even that has been custom designed by the Father.

Perhaps my fear was based on time already spent—the

disappointment of not living up to my own dreams and expectations. No one ever feels the waste of another's life the way she does her own.

I feared change. But change from what? To what? Change is the most consistent part of life. Even granite mountains experience change.

Like Jeremiah, I was commanded to wait if I truly wanted to experience transformation. I learned to love to wait, for it was the process of divine waiting in which I experienced His love.

As we face our fears, we are granted freedom from them. As we enter the darkness, we recognize His Holy light. As we accept dying as a natural part of life, we learn how to live.

Part III
The Spring
A Time to Be Born

Holding Pattern
Voices in the Wind
Hiding Under the Cover

I wait, staring at the clock
Watching the moments of my life unwind
Wondering
Will I ever find rest
Until I find myself in Your arms once again?

Waiting
I awake, suddenly in the night
Trying to find words to make the wrong all turn right
Will I ever find rest
Until I find myself in Your arms once again?

So, I give You my sorrow
You give me Your song
I give You my heart and soul
You give to me meaning and courage to wait.

Yes, she who waits on the Lord shall renew her strength
She shall mount up with wings as eagles
She shall run and not be weary
And she shall walk and not faint.

Be still my soul
Quietly, I wait
As You guide the future
And mend the past.

—MARSHA SPRADLIN

7
Holding Pattern

She is like a tree planted by streams of water,
which yields its fruit in season
and whose leaf does not wither.
Whatever [she] does prospers
(Adapted from Ps. 1:3, NIV).

"Blessed are all who wait for him!"
(Isa. 30:18*b*).

April 1984

"Morning babe! Got your mail. The mail room staff is work-ing overtime trying to keep up with your fan mail. I mean, really, Miss Spradlin. You need to share some of these cards with some of us."

Sherry, the mailwoman, had hardly gotten into my room before the transport "truck" wheeled in to pick me up. The "truck" was what I called the hospital transport bed that came several times a day to take me away for X rays and tests.

"Greetings, Miss M. We've got some good plans for you today. More yummy tests. Say good-bye to Mom and hop aboard."

Our days had become so routine. We had been at the medi-cal center well into the second month. We felt we knew every-one, and they seemed to enjoy their personal relationships with Mother and me.

Each morning I toured the hospital machinery. On many occasions, I felt I had a purpose in being there. The hospital staff had become special. I had now started to adjust to this life-style. It was a world within my own world. Mother, too, was fitting in. While I was out getting the routine tests run each morning, Mother would usually try to catch up on correspondence. She had one real fan that continued to love to get her letters—my daddy:

Hi Honey,
     Can you believe I have been out here over a month? I am just glad we still have her to be with. At the rate she is going, they will never let her out. We are in a holding pattern. No change. Her weight has now locked in at about eighty-three pounds. At least she has not lost. I do feel that this is all firm weight. Dr. Johnson is still running tests. I think he has some ideas that he is not ready to discuss. He makes more sense than all of the others put together.
     Joy, Marsha's boss, came yesterday. Marsha has been so concerned about work and missing three months already. She is now eligible for medical leave. Joy is insisting that she not worry about her job. You know our Marsh!
     We have quite a routine here. I am now a permanent fixture on this hall. I know every nurse and every lab technician. I also know every inch of this hospital. Oh, guess what? I actually drove from the hospital to the condo without getting lost!
     Must go now, honey. Maybe it won't be long until this nightmare will be over. Take care and stay out of trouble.
Love,
Your Number One Wife

Life was not too terribly exciting. There was no real news. The lack of excitement seemed to have a strange effect on me. I had gotten so used to the intensity of the first few weeks that once things relaxed, the blank spaces in my emotions caused me to feel vulnerable or misplaced.

The holding pattern had its own set of temptations and questions. Will life be like this forever? The pain of comparison was the hardest for me. I compared the way life used to be with the way it was and the way it was with the way it might someday be.

I was not aware at the time of the importance of the holding pattern. In many ways, those days of quiet were the most significant in my attempt to recover.

I tried to remember Jeremiah and the wait. This was a time for rest, readjustment of perspective, recognition of purpose, reconciliation of fears and doubts, and renewing my reliance on the Holy Father.

Mornings were better. The evenings were more difficult. I continued to want to hide my fears and emotions, but Mother could often see through my mask. She was extremely sensitive to these ambivalent experiences and mood swings. I could tell she was up to something. She was thinking ahead.

When I returned one day from my routine daily body scan, Mother was waiting.

"OK, Babe, if we're going to lick this thing, we had better get our acts together. What we need is a game plan—a strategy. We need to know we are doing something to make things better. We need something tangible. We have to make our fears, somehow, work for us. I vote that we plan a survival strategy. We can take charge of the fight. I'll be the coach. You're the star player. We can fight anything that tries to sabotage us. After all, you're my kid. Well, are you game?"

I was not aware of it then, but Mom needed the strategy as much as I did. It was a joint venture. And there was no doubt that *she* was the coach. When I blew it, she told me.

"First, we are not in this alone. Have you even stopped to read those cards that came in this morning? I'll bet there are thirty or forty just today. Look at the plants. The gifts. The fruit baskets. Honey, outside these doors are hundreds of people in nearly every state who are praying for you. This pity party every night has got to stop. Starting today, we are going to do one thing each day toward getting you out of here. Besides, I miss your daddy."

So, we started. Together. We really did not know where to start, but we did agree to do something. First, there was the physical aspect.

I had been immobile for nearly two months. The longer I remained that way, the more my muscles, bones, and nerve endings were being damaged. Atrophy had already set in. There was permanent damage. My left leg was partially paralyzed. But I could walk short distances.

Our initial plan was simple. We walked one lap around the floor twice a day. Mother collected books on nutrition and exercise. Each evening, we plotted our strategy for the next day. The walking was painful at first. But Coach Mom encouraged and pushed. Late each evening, she would administer physical therapy to my legs and arms. Eventually, I was able to do leg lifts without assistance. A close friend in Amarillo was a physical therapist; she flew to Dallas to teach us how to do isometrics and other exercises to build remaining muscle tissues.

Socially, Coach Mom insisted that I talk to someone each day with whom I did not have frequent contact. That meant answering at least one phone call daily. Sometimes, she let me count writing a letter as my contact. Frequently, we abducted a wheelchair and escaped to the lobby to visit the gift shop and simply mingle with people. We always stopped to look at the newborn babies and pray at the chapel. In the chapel, we would find prayer request cards submitted by staff members, and my name was almost always listed.

The medical staff was 100 percent in favor of our game plan. We closely documented everything we did for the master chart. "Marsha, you're going down into the who's who of medical journals. We want good records on your recovery," one of the doctors said. My personal fleet of physicians had promised to insert my chest X ray as the centerfold of the 1985 Physician's Desk Reference.

Emotionally, we adopted a philosophy for living. We decided we would not wait for life to return. We would go after it and capture it with the same momentum with which death had tried to capture me. We would live only in the present and reject any attempt to compare life with the way it used to be or maybe could be. "*Now* is the only time there is," Coach Mom insisted.

After the first week of our workout, Mother and Barbara had a surprise reward for me. Early before work, Barb stopped by with a white gift box accented with a blue ribbon. The package was on my bed when I returned from my routine body scan. I loved surprises. I quickly tore through the white paper and flung the top off the box.

"A jogging suit, size 2. It'll fit!"

"Wait, Marsh, there's more." Barbara uncovered the white paper. Little white socks with blue lace. Tears welled up in our eyes and quickly escaped down our cheeks.

"When will I ever get to wear it? I mean, do you think I can ever go home?"

"Hey, who needs to go home to wear that? I think folks around here would welcome the sight of you in something besides that red house coat. Put it on, now."

"In the hospital?"

Mother pulled my Nikes out of the closet.

"Give me one good reason why not. I mean, too many people know you to try to escape this place," insisted Mother.

Instead of putting on the new blue warm-up suit, I decided to go for a total make-over. I had not worn makeup in over a month. I gathered toiletries and my new clothes and escaped to the shower. I stood under the hot water for at least an hour. Mother kept tapping on the door: "Honey, are you OK?"

"Yea, Mom! This is great!"

A nurse came in to take my blood pressure and listen to my ticker. "Where is she?"

"Just wait a minute, Cindy."

"Mrs. Spradlin, are you letting that girl take a hot shower by herself?"

"Oh, yes! I taught her how to wash behind her ears last year," Mother laughed. She enjoyed joking with Cindy.

"But, Mrs. Spradlin, she could faint or even . . ."

"Yes, Cindy, but she could die out here, too. At least she will be clean!"

Cindy smiled.

"Cindy, we're not afraid of dying anymore. Actually, it's living that scares us. But I'd rather see her enjoy being than dreading becoming."

Cindy took the breakfast tray. Evidently, she shared our little escapade with the nursing staff. When I stepped out of the bathroom, all decked out in my blue jogging outfit, not to mention the Nikes and socks, I felt like I was sixteen again and going to the prom. The entire nursing staff had packed into my room. They were cheering and laughing and making cracks. "Go for it, babe! We're right behind you." Mother and Barbara simply smiled and exchanged hand squeezes.

"OK, Marsh, are you ready for your maiden voyage around the floor?"

We slowly walked, arm in arm. Not only did we walk, this time we investigated halls, doors, storage rooms, and other places off limits for patients. But after all, we considered ourselves residents.

Unfortunately, or maybe fortunately, we ran into Dr. Gonzales.

"What is this? Shouldn't you be in a wheelchair?

"Come on, Dr. G."

Just to make a scene, he took my blood pressure right in the hallway.

"You're good for five more minutes, then you, Cinderella, had better get in your little cottage before your Nikes are seized."

We laughed and continued our investigation. Over the next ten days, walking became my therapy. I learned to recognize the importance of listening to myself and my body for instructions. Actually, I am now convinced that the instructions came as answered prayer.

We learned later that the physical activity strengthened the heart muscles that had already undergone enormous stress and atrophy. The valves could be strengthened through repetitive physical activity. Likewise, diet became a priority in my survival strategy. We later learned that this was one of the most positive things I could have done. Sugar is a stimulant—not good for patients with funny heart beats. Fat—well, I needed it, but not that kind. Instead, protein was identified as a muscle builder and a good source of energy.

Spiritually, my therapy was waiting and trusting. But during the wait, I struggled to learn the meaning of some of God's greatest truths. To be still and know God, for example, Mother and I had devotions daily, both privately and together. She loved to read. As she read, she shared. She encouraged me to write what I could not say. We prayed, we cried, we loved. We knew we were recipients of thousands of prayers across the United States.

Socially, my therapy came into action as Mrs. Powell, my morning nurse, told me about Karen, another patient. I shall never forget her. Mrs. Powell encouraged me to give her hope.

"Marsha, please, I want you to visit her. She is just two doors down. I think she is giving up."

Karen was near death. She was twenty-one years old and beautiful, even though she only weighed ninety-four pounds. She was hooked up to some rather familiar medical gadgets.

I walked past her room and looked in, then decided I couldn't invade her privacy.

"Mrs. Powell, I can't. Look at me. I'm smaller than Karen. I am eighty-four pounds on a good day, and I am probably a lot taller than she is."

Mrs. Powell all but scolded me.

"Yes, look at you! You are a walking miracle. So far, you have lived to tell about it. Karen needs hope and encouragement. I just thought you could help. After all, you give us all hope and courage. You're the talk of this hospital. You are a miracle. God knows Karen needs a miracle right now."

I dug deep for the courage to visit Karen. Quietly, I crept toward her bed. I thought she was asleep, so I tried to walk softly. My Nikes squeaked on the shiny tile floor loud enough to awaken her. She looked dead. She was a dim reflection of who she had been—a shadow of herself. I was unable to speak at first. I simply took her hand. Tears stole my sight.

"Karen, I live a couple doors down. I just wanted to meet my new neighbor. After all, I have been here a long time. I thought I could, maybe, show you some of the ropes around here."

Karen said nothing. She looked strange to me. I was scared something was wrong.

"I have to go. Karen, I love you. Please don't stop trying to live. Please, Karen!"

I ran out of the room to escape my own feelings of devastation. I managed to get to my bathroom. I was flooded with doubts, depression, and darts. The pit of my stomach felt as if all of my fear had settled there. I looked in the mirror as I pulled back my hair.

"Is that me? Do I look like Karen? Oh, dear God! I do. Am I dying, too?"

Karen became my personal project. I prayed for her and loved her. On my daily walks, I would stop briefly to cheer her on. I never got to know Karen very well. Less than a week after my first visit, I found her room empty. Karen had not been as lucky as I was. She had died.

Reflections on Rest

Waiting, resting, patience! Each play an active part in any holding pattern. Each are profoundly common. They are their own rewards.

Life itself seems to rub against the grain of these virtues. Nature abhors a vacuum. Where there is an empty space, something slips in making rest almost impossible. If anything is removed, something must fill it. This philosophy of life keeps us from waiting. We are doers. We must make it happen. We must be in control. But the question is, can we rest and have patience while we actively participate in God's plan? Or, are waiting, resting, and patience simply passive? Is there such a thing as active waiting?

What is rest? Rest is realizing God is in control. Resting is not the same as doing nothing. Rest is doing something— resting. Rest is not to be confused with physical inactivity. It is more. It is emotional, spiritual, and absolutely essential for healing of any kind.

Rest is readjustment to the way life is. It encourages us not to compare life to the way it has always been. Instead, it encourages us to see through new eyes—eyes of compassion.

Rest is reconciliation. It urges us to let go of our hurts and fears.

Rest is responsibility. It motivates us to take action. Any action is better than nothing. But we can't confuse this positive action with *not* resting.

Rest is recognition. It reminds us to see who we are and Whose we are.

Every opportunity to rest gives us more energy to live. By resting, we have time to define our purpose. Lack of purpose is a waste and creates a human vacuum. Rest, then, brings purpose, and purpose defines our productivity.

We were not made simply to exist, but to exist for something: to have dominion over all the earth (Gen. 1:26). We are to be creative.

This divine call to creativity, productivity, industry, and conquest burns in the soul of each of us. Take away our opportunity to fulfill this call, and life loses its rest, and the vacuum settles in. Despair comes not so much from being deprived of more but from not being able to use what we already have. By simply resting, the light of dawn comes to those of us who could have felt hedged in.

The wind is blowing again;
Its voice calls my name,
It sings,
It whispers,
It knows me well;
I have come to call it my friend.

No! I am not afraid that it is blowing again;
I have nailed down the broken parts.
The storm may come,
The tempest may rise,
But the voice of the wind will forever be my friend.

As the rushing wind of Your spirit breezes through my soul
May it push me forward;
May I run and not be weary,
Walk and not faint,
Glide in the power of Your wind.

Only then, kind Father,
Will Your sweet spirit of joy rush in,
Carrying me on to a new day,
Giving bright hope for all of my tomorrows.

—MARSHA SPRADLIN

8
Voices in the Wind

He makes winds his messengers,
flames of fire his servants (Ps. 104:4).

He who doubts is like a wave of the sea, blown and tossed by the wind
(Jas. 1:6b).

The wind blows wherever it pleases.
You hear its sound, but you cannot tell
where it comes from or where it is going.
So it is with everyone born of the Spirit
(John 3:8).

Late April 1984

The rain tapped rhythmically on the window, creating gloomy but tranquil effects. The wind brought another storm into the Dallas/Fort Worth area. It had rained for days.

We were now launching the sixth week at the medical center. Neither the rain nor my extended time in the hospital made the atmosphere sedate. Instead, my mind and spirit were preoccupied with a rehearsal; the reward of a correct performance would be my freedom. I was convinced that this was the time to exert myself. I wanted to go home, desperately. But winning Dr. Kennedy over to my perspective would be more difficult than anything so far. I knew that I myself must be perfectly convinced, sure, secure! So, I rehearsed.

There was no reason to stay in the hospital, I felt. I could not imagine a test that had not been performed. I could not think of a corner of the hospital that I had not explored at least once.

I also knew that the state of my health was no better than it was when I was admitted nearly six weeks earlier. In fact, it was worse. But, I maintained, if I am not getting better, why not *not* get better at home!

My vital signs were locked into a very below-normal level. My weight had stabilized at eighty-two and a half—lower than it had been when I was admitted in March. The game plan, as far as the physicians were concerned, was to terminate all tests, except for body scans. I had been instructed to "stay on the hall." I had gotten brave and taken a few trips off my floor—and gotten caught! I needed constant monitoring. But I could do most of that myself.

It seemed like this could go on forever! The more I thought about it, the stronger I wanted to go home.

"When Dr. K. comes in today, I will just tell him. After all, I am an adult. I can decide. They can't just keep me here."

It was Sunday. Dr. Kennedy made rounds late on Sunday. I reminded myself that he was at church and was supposed to be praying for me.

Even though I anticipated every tap on the door to be his, his arrival caught me off guard.

"Happy Sunday to you! Did you see my church service on TV?"

Before I could answer, he asked, "Where's the coach?"

"Oh, she went down the hall for a newspaper. She likes to get the coupons from the Sunday paper. I am really kind of glad she is not here. I need to talk. Wait a minute, I wrote down what I want to say."

I had outlined all the reasons why I should be released.

He propped his foot on the chair next to my bed and did not appear to be in a hurry. He was ready to hear me out.

"I think it's time for me to go home. Now before you get too excited, please listen. I've spent all morning on this speech."

Dr. Kennedy shifted, as if to put up a guard. He was preparing his defense.

"First, you said I need complete rest. Now, come on. One does not rest here. Nurses are in every fifteen minutes wanting to take something out of me or put something in. The sticking, knocking, thumping—you know what goes on around here. And, then there is nighttime. I have actually been awakened in the middle of the night by nurses trying to find out if I was asleep. Hospitals are simply not for sick people.

"Second, the food. You said I could have anything I wanted and plenty of it. I need good food. Enough said!

"I have some more reasons, but I can't think right now.

"Oh, yes, this room needs to go to someone else. I have had it long enough. Besides, I've tied up your life—as well as six other doctors—for months. You guys need to get to work."

Dr. Kennedy tapped his pen nervously against his leg and walked to the window. He stared into the stormy rain outside for minutes. He slowly turned and ran his fingers through his hair. I knew he was thinking when he ran his fingers through his hair. He always did that.

"Marsha, I nearly blew it with you. I should have put you in here months before you nearly died. I let you talk me out of it, but not again. I cannot allow it. You think you feel good. But compared to what? Your blood pressure is not high enough to even give you enough support to walk across this room, much less run around the hospital. I simply don't know what is keeping you alive. I don't know, either, what is trying to sabotage you.

"Look in the mirror. You are 5'7", and you weigh eighty-two pounds dripping wet and full of IVs. My dog weighs more than that dry and dehydrated. You are still having terrible blood reports. Here's one."

He thrust the paper into my hand. The numbers meant nothing to me. But I knew.

"I can't fix the funny heart rhythms right now. The beta blockers would make your blood pressure drop even lower. You're a mess. If you are not real careful, you will be on a respirator the rest of your life. And you know about the white blood count. You are still in the low twos. It looks bad—real bad. There is not a doctor in the world that can bring that count up. Your body's immune system has simply shut down. I can't let you go home. Not now."

"When?"

"I can't answer that. There are simply too many unknowns. What I don't know scares me. What I do know is causing me to lose weight."

"There is one option. Mayo Clinic. I talked with them today. They have agreed to take you. They are very selective but have agreed that you could be a candidate for some research. That will mean more tests, but, at this point, that is your only option."

My enthusiasm began to sink as it was submerged in disappointment. I felt like a child being scolded for something I did not do. I felt victimized again. I felt the storm rushing in.

"Dr. Kennedy, do you pray for me?"

He picked up my hand and gently squeezed it.

"Every day, Marsha. Every day!" He blinked quickly to avoid tears.

"I will stay as long as you will pray for me and promise not to give up on me. I need to know you haven't given up."

He did not give up, but he did give in—a little. He was leaving for a two-week study trip to Hawaii. Before departing the hospital that afternoon, he came by for a final good-bye and to give me something.

"Surprise! This, young lady, is good for a two-hour trip outside these hospital walls. You can leave—but for two hours only. Remember two things: Come back, or you're grounded! And don't even think about going anywhere near germs." He smiled and quickly left.

Mother returned moments later with excitement painted over her face.

"Well, honey, we are not going to Hawaii, but what about White Rock Lake?"

We called Barbara, and she rushed to the hospital emergency entrance to meet us. As we drove away, a familiar feeling of freedom came over me. It was refreshing. It reminded me of walking barefoot on the grass after wearing shoes all winter.

It was strange, but familiar; happy, but sad; exciting, but a little frightening.

White Rock Lake was not too far from the hospital. The rain had ceased, but the wind was still blowing. The air was very brisk. Barbara and I had spent many special Sunday afternoons riding bicycles around the lake and picnicking. Remembering how it used to be suddenly flooded my mind, washing away the joy. The pain of comparison—I had come to know it well.

Mom, Barb, and I found a picnic table beneath a little tree— there are no big trees in Texas. Together we sat, shoulder to shoulder, scrunched together to stay warm. Barbara had brought a small cushion from her car. I could not sit on anything harder than an egg-crate mattress.

We did not feel a need to speak. We simply sat watching the sailboats maneuver. How strange it was that each boat went in such separate paths and directions within the same body of water. But each one was powered by the same source—the wind. I could see the boats, but I could not see the source of their power. I could only feel its effects. At times, my tiny body felt like it would be lifted off the table by the sudden puffs of wind. As I watched the boats I realized that most of the sailors could not explain how it all worked—the power and the sails. Nor could they predict when the powerful source of energy would be available again. Each sailor simply had to wait. No one had an edge on the wind.

The wind treated each sailor equally. Its power was available to all. It was the sailor that made the difference. Some were not prepared and were caught with their sails down, missing their chance to take advantage of the powerful gusts. Some were frightened by a sudden surge; they froze and missed the opportunity to move forward. Some were crippled—their boats sank. Others struggled to learn how to maneuver the sails; they were inexperienced sailors but willing to learn even—even though that meant taking chances. Perhaps these were the ones who eventually became "real sailors." Finally, some were fully pre-

pared. They were seasoned sailors. They could move forward
with the same source of power that frustrated and sank the
others. What did it all mean—the voices in the wind?

> He makes winds his messengers,
> flames of fire his servants
> (Ps 104:4).

Maybe I, too, could use the power from this unknown source
—the illness? It had tried to sabotage me and sink me. Could
I gain power from something I had been interpreting as negative? Could I choose how to use the power? Or would I be
frightened, frustrated, and even caught off guard? All of those
responses could sink me.

Could I wait patiently, sitting tightly in my little boat, listening for this voice in the wind, trusting that at the perfect
moment I could move forward? I realized I must be prepared
but willing to wait. I must be willing to learn. And I must be
willing to nearly sink at times. I must know that I can always
get back in the boat and try again. Sooner or later, I will learn
how to use the wind as my power. Could I remember that
when the wind blows the hardest, I can move the greatest
distance? Only I can decide how I will set my sails. Maybe I
should consider sailing school!

We returned to the medical center only moments before the
curfew. I was exhausted. I realized that Dr. Kennedy had used
psychology on me. I was weaker than I thought. He had proven
his point. But I still wanted to go home.

After Dr. Kennedy left, I was assigned to Dr. Gonzales.
There was a mix-up on my chart—a marvelous mix-up, as far
as I was concerned.

The morning after Dr. Kennedy left for Hawaii, Dr. Gonzales, who was Cuban, walked into my room speaking Spanish.

"You look happy, Dr. Gonzales, but I can't understand a
word you are saying. I don't know why that should bother me;
I have not understood too much you have said in English."

"Today you will enjoy understanding. You are leaving!"

"Not Mayo. Please, Dr. Gonzales."

"Who said anything about Mayo? I am sending you home. But before you get too excited, there are a couple of things we need to agree on. First, you are not better. I am saying that because most people think going home means being well. You are not well. You are very sick, in fact. For that reason, you are grounded. I don't want you to go outside the Dallas city limits."

"No problem! I just want to go to North Dallas. Forest Lane to be exact."

"Actually, this will have to be evaluated almost daily. Here's the plan. Every other day, you will have to come to Dr. Kennedy's office at 10:00 AM. Absolutely no excuses. On any one of those days, we may have to readmit you. If you miss one appointment, I will personally come after you. You are on probation.

"We want to do blood work regularly. We can't seem to fix your problem, but we can watch it. Did Dr. Kennedy explain to you about your white blood count? Your bone marrow still refuses to manufacture cells. Your count would put most of us in ICU. But you are tolerating it well. Remember, no germs. I have prescriptions for antibiotics. This is just for protection.

"One other thing. Watch that weight. One pound down, I want a phone call. Two pounds down, pack your toothbrush and, of course, that red robe.

"For the pain, well, all we can do is give you drugs. Be careful. They are addictive.

"I want you to sleep. I will also write a prescription to help you.

"We will hold off on the beta blockers until your weight gets up. I am a little afraid of that right now.

"Good luck. At ninety pounds, we will party!"

Mother and I celebrated by having a card-taking-down party. Over the nearly sixty days I had been there, I had continued to receive cards, letters, and telegrams as well as prayer-grams and gifts. Every inch of the room and door was covered with love. These expressions reminded me of friends needing to demonstrate their concern. But they also reminded me of the pain I had endured.

Mother got several large boxes for the cards. One by one, we removed them from the wall. As the blue-and-beige wallpaper became apparent, my memories of March 13 became apparent as well. I could hear Pat, "Look Marsh, blue-and-beige wallpa-per, just like your condo. You must have connections to have gotten this room." I had connections, but not the kind Pat was referring to.

"Mother, can't we throw these away? I am OK now. Besides, where will I put them at home?"

"One day, honey, you will wish you had these."

I said nothing, only to humor her. But quietly inside, I made plans to destroy them. I just could not be sick anymore.

As we packed my stuff, I began to feel that maybe I was not as ready to leave as I thought I was. I was not emotionally prepared to say good-bye to the only place my insecure body had identified as safe.

As we tore each card off the wall, I felt a tearing inside. The reality of the unknown began to haunt me. I couldn't see what was next on the journey. If I just had a clue. Will I get better? Will I always stay just like this? Will I get worse? Will I ever work again or be productive and creative? I gazed out my window as I had on many occasions before when I needed to think. I remembered the wind, the power. I could see the storm, the clouds, and even hear thunder. I knew that my hopes could easily be washed away at any moment. But then I remembered Jeremiah. I must learn the urgency of waiting patiently. And, as I wait, I must redirect my fear of the unknown to a powerful life directed by faith in the Source of all power. Only faith can move me forward. But like the wind, faith is invisible. So was my fate. I couldn't hold it or embrace it. I couldn't see it. I could only see the results.

Leaving was the biggest step of faith so far. I tried to remember that He had been a shelter for me. He had been a sanctuary from the storm. He would always be a refuge for me.

Saying good-bye was difficult. I had come to love the hospital staff. On the day of my release, many came by to express their love and encourage me onward. No one knew what the future held, but we knew that we had all participated in a miracle. Each person brought to my mind special memories of who they were and where we had been together:

Cindy—the nurse who mothered me and loved my mother.

Debbie—I shall never forget her, the young Catholic nurse in ICU. She believed in me when no one else did. I knew I would love her forever. We spent the darkest hours of my life together. I will always remember Debbie, hours after she was supposed to go off duty, tapping away on the computer. Later she told me she was afraid to leave. "I was afraid that if I left you, I would never see you again. You were my friend, and you were dying."

Ruth—the floor supervisor who let me break nearly every rule.

Susan—the IV supervisor. She was affectionately known as my private vampire. Ready and willing, Susan was on the spot to take my blood. After my veins collapsed she rigged a device so she would not have to go through the painful procedure to retread my veins. "I know it is sort of trite, Marsha, but this does hurt me more than you."

Brad—the ambulance driver. I barely remember him from the March 13th experience. What made him special were his frequent visits, even when the "no visitors" sign was posted.

Lisa—the staff dietitian. We spent hours calculating calories and scratching our heads. "How can you lose weight on 6,000 calories a day? You have more spunk than I do."

Bob—the chaplain. We were friends in graduate school.

Now we were friends from the bonding that comes from sharing some of life's rarest moments.

Beth—one special X-ray technician. I visited her daily. "What are you doing back here? I thought yesterday's picture was good enough for the medical journal's centerfold."

I entered the medical center without a toothbrush. I left with more than two carloads of cards, plants, fruit baskets, an ice chest, and coffee pot. Mom and I were like a couple of college roommates going home at the end of the term. We felt surely we had received some type of degree. We had certainly taken enough tests.

Driving away was almost like leaving home. Fear built. But I was determined not to show it. This is a happy day. Smile, make them think you're happy. Smile, make them think things are going fine. I must be strong. How can I ever get strong if I am not strong enough to be strong?

I had thought very little about the March 13 episode until the day of my release. Now, on this special day, I was reminded of Dr. Gonzales's conversation. I was not well, but I wanted so much to be. I wanted to convince the world, but I was not convinced. I knew Mother wasn't either.

Fear haunted me as we slowly walked up the stairs to my condo. Memories of being carted on a stretcher by unknown men flooded my thoughts. I stopped on the stairs and bent into a tightly curled wad. Tears flooded my eyes as memories flooded my emotions. For most, being released meant the storm was over. But I was starting to feel the wind blow hard again. *I must hold on and not abort my ship. The voices in the wind—I must listen to my pain. For as I listen, I shall learn something magnificent.*

Reflections on Trust

I had thought that seeing was believing. But I came to realize that believing was seeing! I did not know where I was going. But I did know who was going with me. And, if I was going with Him, I had to revise my attitude toward who He was. I had to see Him and Him alone, not myself, my lack, limitations, or fear.

"Take no thought for your life or for your body." In other words, I must not think about those things of which I had been thinking—myself.

What was God doing?

Soon I learned that He would not tell me. For telling me would only cause me to lose sight of who He was and redirect my focus back toward myself. He simply insisted that I focus on who He was.

Leaving the medical center was "going out on a limb." It was the perfect opportunity for Him to teach me that only through believing could I see where I had gone and why.

I can see that clearly now. But during those days, I had not yet learned to see through His eyes. The joy of discovery!

Yes, believing is seeing. It is called *faith*. The question continues to be, "Do I trust you, Lord?"

Humility—I feel stripped to the core
Barren, naked
Where is my dignity?
Where is my cover?
Why am I a prisoner to their cross-examination
I want to hide
But nowhere can I go that I am not there.

Forever I have been enslaved with foolish vanity
But now, I see that such pride was not Your plan for me.
How else can they see your light burn bright
Unless I make my life transparent?
Can you create a heart so pure that I have nothing to hide

Oh, Father, may my life become an open book
For others to read
Let them know me for who I am
I am Yours
You are mine
Open my heart to realize
That they need to see You
Through humility in me.

—Marsha Spradlin

9
Hiding Under the Cover

In the same way, the Spirit helps us in our weakness.
We do not know what we ought to pray,
but the Spirit himself intercedes for us with groans
that words cannot express
(Rom. 8:26).

The light is short because of darkness
(Job 17:12, KJV).

Late April-May 1984

Light spilled into the room, splitting the darkness. I hid my eyes to avoid it.

"Arise, sleeper. Awake. Be fully alive!"

It was Mother again. She stood in my bedroom doorway holding a cup of coffee and decked out for walking. She was wearing her "Coach Mom" shirt. I had given it to her shortly after being released from the hospital. After all, she had always wanted to be a coach. In my opinion, she had earned the position.

"Up and shoes on! Let's go! Time for a lap or two around the parking lot before the sun takes over the morning. I know rest is important, honey, but walking is essential. Remember what the physical therapist told us about atrophy."

I slowly threw my rail-like legs to the side of the bed. Atrophy had definitely set in. My arms and legs, as well as fingers, had lost muscle tissue. I had difficulty not only walking but even holding a fork. So, therapy became important. We walked and ate.

Getting up in the morning was not easy. I was highly sedated. The intent was quality sleep. I had accomplished that. As soon as I was fully awake, I simply took another pill and was out again. Life was not that bad. I could hide my fears and even the pain, to a large degree, under the covers in my darkened room. I did not have to think, feel, listen, or deal with the reality within the walls of my condo or within the walls of my own narrow life.

I knew that if I was going to convince Mother that I was fine, I was going to have to stop this Sleeping Beauty routine and act like a responsible adult.

The first days home were far from restful. The telephone rang constantly. Friends with whom I had not talked in years were finally able to express their concern. The "no visitors" sign hanging outside my hospital door was not hanging on Forest Lane. A string of visitors stopped by—some announced and some unexpected. I often felt invaded. I knew I shouldn't have these feelings.

I was a private person. In my "old" life, I seldom left the bathroom without a full face of makeup. Now, suddenly, I felt on display. While I realized people did not mean to seem obsessed with my lack of figure, it was obvious to me that they were shocked. Often, I would crack a joke to break the trance of their discomfort.

Mother and Barb become hypersensitive to my needs. They tried to protect me from the infinite string of phone calls and even screen the visitors.

After several days at home, it suddenly occurred to me that Mother could not continue to live with me forever. I was thirty years old. The nightmare could go on infinitely. She had a life to live and a business to manage. Yet this was not a decision either of us could make alone. We had to make it together, yet separately. How could she leave with so many uncertainties? But how could she continue to stay with such uncertainties.

What hope and certainties did we have? None. But what hope and certainties do any of us have? Absolutely none. I started praying that I would know when to initiate the suggestion that Mother return to Alabama. Until then, I decided to wait.

The trips back to the medical center for the blood work and body scan were strange. I dreaded returning only two days after my mistaken and artificial release. But I looked forward to it, too. Part of the agreement meant wearing the exact same clothing on every visit. I am sure the hospital staff got tired of my size-two jogging suit. But this ensured a more accurate weight reading. Every ounce counted. Each could mean either life or death in the balances.

The first visits were happy ones, even though blood tests and scans are never happy ordeals. With each visit came more questions and no answers. More documentation was done. I went home with a brown paper bag stuffed with cans of liquid supplement to help with weight gain. For the first weeks, I was stable. I did not lose or gain. This became a cue to talk with Mother.

On the way home from the hospital one day I got the nerve to say it:

"Don't you think you should be thinking about going home? We both know this cannot go on forever. We just can't live this way." Tears once again began to steal my sight. We both knew it was time.

I realized just how much she had given me. She had not left me for five minutes in over two months. I had not spent that much time with her since I was a preschooler. She had focused her every thought and her total energy toward me. Every part of me wanted her to stay.

In many ways I felt like a young child entering school on the first day. I remembered the first grade—knowing that I wanted to go to school because I was six years old. Six-year-olds are supposed to want to go to school. But deep inside I was scared. As a six-year-old, I remembered not wanting to leave her, but I went anyway, holding the tears back and watching other kids cry. They, too, missed their moms. I remembered feeling that

I couldn't wait until I grew up. It shouldn't hurt then. I was wrong! In many ways, I was six years old again. In many ways, it hurt more. Yes, I was entering school again. And, yes, I had to go alone.

Two days later, Daddy arrived to take my mother and his wife home. We spent most of Saturday afternoon just being together. Neither of us felt the need to entertain. Mother stocked my cabinets with groceries. Dad did a few handyman-type chores. Early the next morning, we said good-bye. I remember very little about those moments. The pain was obviously too intense. How could we adequately say good-bye and bring a closure to this experience? My heart could hear their hearts as we embraced.

I remember the hours after they left. It was Easter Sunday. I wanted to spend it in church, next to Mother, Daddy, Larry, and Teresa—just as always. But *always* was no longer real. I spent Easter alone for the first time ever.

Rather than putting on a pretty Easter outfit, I put on my only piece of clothing that fit—the size-two blue warm-ups and top. Instead of driving to church to worship, I went to a jogging track nearby. There, with my Bible and notebook, I read the Easter story. I read how He was abused, cursed, and accused of things He did not do; how His body ached and how His hands, too, bled. He did not despise His accusers. He loved them. I read:

> For a little while longer the light is among you. Walk while you have the light, that darkness may not overtake you; he who walks in the darkness does not know where he goes. While you have the light, believe in the light, in order that you may become sons of light (John 12:35-36, NASB).

> I am the true vine, and My Father is the vinedresser. Every branch in Me that does not bear fruit, He takes away; and every branch that bears fruit, He prunes it, that it may bear more fruit. You are already clean because of the word which I have spoken to you. Abide in Me, and I in you. As the branch cannot bear

fruit of itself, unless it abides in the vine, so neither can you, unless you abide in Me. I am the vine, you are the branches; he who abides in Me, and I in him, he bears much fruit; for apart from Me you can do nothing. If anyone does not abide in Me, he is thrown away as a branch, and dries up; and they gather them, and cast them into the fire, and they are burned. If you abide in Me, and My words abide in you, ask whatever you wish, and it shall be done for you. By this is My Father glorified that you bear much fruit, and so prove to be My disciples (John 15:1-8, NASB).

I thought. I prayed. I marveled on that Easter Sunday. The sun had risen and nearly set. I was still sitting on the park bench considering the meaning of the verses I had read a hundred times. But it seemed new and fresh. I remembered Lamentations 3:22-23: "The Lord's lovingkindnesses indeed never cease, For His compassions never fail. They are new every morning" (NASB).

Perhaps my morning had come. The Son had risen and was now dwelling inside my life. I had been pruned.

All that I need, He gives just in time. Otherwise, I would not have made it through this first day on my own without the rushing energy of His Spirit.

When I returned to my condo, the phone was ringing. I barely made it in time.

"Hi, Honey. Daddy and I are home."

"Already? You just left!"

"Just left? That was twelve hours ago."

"Mother, you would not believe my good day."

"It should have been good. Daddy and I prayed for you all day." By now, our eyes had been seasoned by many tears. I could tell Mother was crying. "Good night, honey. I will call you tomorrow. No! You call me when you get back from Dr. Kennedy's. I want a report. Remember, 10:00 AM."

"I'll remember, coach! Love you, too."

I thought that night of the Father's love—loving enough to

let His only Son go. I thought of my own parents—loving enough to let me go.

I wish every day could have been like that one. They were not. I continued to hide under the cover of my own self-deception. Fear continued to rip through my spirit. But I was unwilling to admit to anyone the degree of my pain.

The routine began to form. Routines gave way to habits: every-other-day checkups, eating every hour, sleeping as much as possible. All of my habits were necessary and inno-cent. But innocence does not always reap innocence. Such was the drug therapy.

My doctors had prescribed a class-four narcotic for pain. In addition, I was taking sleeping pills, sedatives, and a host of other "legal" agents to make me better. The physical pain became extreme after about the fourth week out of the hospi-tal. There was no explanation for it. All I knew was that it seemed impossible that anybody could absorb so much an-guish. I was not aware that that degree of pain even existed. The pain became routine. Daily it greeted me like a thief steal-ing my rest and hope. Accompanying the pain was fever. Each day, around 9:00 or so in the morning, my body began to feel like it was breaking into small pieces. The pain may have been there around the clock, with the nightly sedatives temporarily camouflaging it.

I had always been quick to judge those who could not handle pain. That was before I learned the definition of it. Regardless, I knew only one thing: nothing had prepared me to endure such torture. I had to escape.

I took cold baths many times each day to lower the fever. Often I would empty entire trays of ice into the already-cold water hoping to make it colder. The pain and fever frightened me. I found myself sleeping day and night with my door un-locked. I feared getting worse and no one being able to get to me in time. I began to live once again in my own prison of fear.

I knew that the prescribed drugs were habit-forming. I took

precautions. I broke the already-small pills in half for a while. Then, no longer did I feel their effects. Soon, one whole pill was not enough, then two. Then I craved them. I did not want the drugs, or the euphoric feelings they manifested, but the escape. No longer did I feel the pain; I felt nothing. I was not afraid. I was not alive, either.

How could this, too, be happening to me? Questions consumed my thoughts: How do spiritual eyes go bad? When do deceptions infiltrate the mind? It happened so slowly, but so quickly. It was innocent, but intentional. I felt trapped. I did not cause my pain. I only wanted relief. I did not ask for fear. I only wanted freedom.

Fear was always more intense when the scales indicated a decline—regardless how small. One morning, I weighed in at home—part of my routine. I couldn't believe it. I had lost two pounds. I remembered Dr. Gonzales's promise to readmit me if I lost two pounds. I had always been considered creative. That day I knew I really had to put my creative energy to work. "Where there is a will, there is a way." I had the will.

In my kitchen was a canister of several hundred pennies. I had been collecting them for some unknown reason. They came in handy. I carefully stacked them and covered the stack in masking tape—an appropriate name! I then found some hospital arm tourniquets used for blood tests and injections. I used these to strap the rolls of pennies onto the calves of my legs. I then concealed them by pulling my blue knee socks over the artificial weight. My blue jogging pants gave me the added cover. I was ready.

Before leaving for the hospital, I ate two cups of Jello and drank volumes of water to give my weight an extra boost. Anything to make myself weigh more. "Ah, bananas! Yes, they weigh something." I ate two!

Wouldn't you know this had to be the day that Dr. Kennedy had an emergency. So I had to wait. The pennies strapped to my legs began to feel tight. The Jello and volumes of water began to feel explosive inside my tiny bladder. I thought I wouldn't make it.

Soon, I weighed in. That was always the first procedure before the blood work and other tests.

"Well, Marsha, congratulations. You are up one ounce today. You must have had rocks in your pockets."

How did he know?

Relief! Guilt! Pain! I quickly excused myself before any of the other blood tests were done.

As I left the hospital, the guilt was more pronounced than the relief. How could I do such a thing? I was too scared not to. Even though I had pulled the wool over Dr. Kennedy's eyes, I knew that my weight was down. I knew what that could mean.

The manipulation of the weight was not nearly as concerning as the manipulation of my feelings. I had opened the medicine cabinet too frequently. Was I becoming addicted to my only source of help for the physical pain? Were the codeine and morphine becoming an escape that camouflaged the emotional pain as well? Did I rationalize? *Many people with far less pain were far more dependent than I,* I thought.

As I forced myself to recognize the building dependency, I tried to cut down. I soon realized that facing this, much less overcoming it, would take far more energy and courage than I had.

Once again, I remembered the wind, my tiny ship, and the voice. I must capture the wind by first accepting it. There is no other way to fight. The wind must be on my side. I can't allow it to blow against me. Where is the wind when I need it? I remembered that all I ran from I would eventually run to. Where is the voice in the wind? I will, I must, I have to set my sail and wait.

So, with the Source giving me strength and courage, I opened each bottle. Slowly, I poured the contents into a large bowl. The colorful pills looked almost like candy. They were for some, but not for me. I had a greater Power within. Quickly, while I still had the courage, I flushed the narcotics down the toilet. As each one disappeared, I embraced the wind with humility.

Reflections on Humility

I had equated my worth with what I did or how well I did it. If I did not do it anymore, then I was not good anymore. I did not realize that God's love for me did not depend upon me, my actions, or my lack of actions. I did not know that it was OK to be weak and defeated. It was OK to not know how to handle pain.

I also thought I was supposed to figure things out for myself and then make them better. I could not figure out this experience. I was a wounded warrior. I did not know how to run home as a wounded warrior. Running home does not mean a lack of faith. It means faith in the One you have identified as the source of your help.

I wish I had known then that it really was OK to go home, running to the Father, when I was wounded. It does not matter to the Father why I fall down; what does matter is who picks me up and how.

As I accept my defeats, pain, and fears for what they are and are not, I come to know myself. I free myself to no longer hide from the only One who really knows me.

Feeling pain and defeat is not lack of faith. It is an opportunity to practice faith. As I share my fears and pain with the Father, I recognize that only He knows me well enough to fix my broken wings. It is only then that I can rise above humiliation.

Part IV
The Summer
A Time to Reap

Dignity Denied
Designing My Destiny
Effects of the Son

There is pain in my heart
My dignity has been denied
I've been torn apart
Covered in fear
Lost in my pride
Trying to hide.

Why do I feel so unsure
Accused, abused, bruised.

Yes, Lord, I have been known to compromise
But I could never truly live outside Your will

So, living God,
Consuming fire
Make Your will my desire
And take my life
Give it the dignity You desire
As You mold it like clay in Your hands
Refine me
That I might shine as Your purest gold

—Marsha Spradlin

10
Dignity Denied

Clothe yourselves with humility toward one another, because,
"God opposes the proud but gives grace to the humble."
Humble yourselves, therefore, under God's mighty hand,
that he may lift you up in due time
(1 Pet. 5:5).

May-June 1984

Seeing my reflection in a mirror reminded me of the trick mirrors at the state fair. As a child, I enjoyed seeing what I would look like if I were tall, short, fat, or even skinny. I was a skinny child. Looking even skinnier used to be funny. But now, seeing my unclothed reflection in my full-length mirror was far from funny. Nothing I saw seemed like me. I was confident that if I had been at the fair, people would pay admission to stare at this freak figure. I had to stop looking in the mirror. Feelings of horror began to steal my breath. I had refused to see—until now. I simply would not look. Each glance now lashed out at my self-esteem and confidence.

My dignity had been denied *physically*. For months, I had slept on a foam egg crate to ease the pain. These mats were designed for persons who could not tolerate anything touching their bodies for very long. My second place of escape was a special padded pallet in my small living room. The cushion in my car allowed me to ride short distances. But soon I found myself not wanting to go anywhere. In the hospital and at home, I felt safe, protected from the germs. But the fear of germs infecting my childlike body was not what made me feel vulnerable. It was the reality of my rejection.

Self-confidence was once mine. I never had to pay much attention to my body. Weight control was never a problem. I was fit, healthy, and usually noticed in a crowd. I seldom had trouble getting dates or attention.

I was not prepared for the physical changes. They did not happen suddenly. Just as the night seldom begins abruptly, the deprivation of my body came gradually—like fall turning into winter. As each leaf lets go of the branch—one by one—giving way to winter, my physical decline—ounce by ounce—gave way to a declining self-concept. But suddenly I noticed it—like a sudden rush of wind before the first winter storm of the season.

I was a victim, I felt. I obviously had identified my "good" with my body. But physical security was no longer yielding dividends. My body was not a good investment.

My dignity was denied *socially*. As long as I was at the hospital, I felt safe. I was sick. Sick people are supposed to look strange and weak. But soon I learned that the world is not prepared to deal with people who look, act, and even feel different from the norm. Even well-intentioned people did not know what to do with me, much less what to say or how to say it.

My dignity was denied *mentally*. There must be an unwritten rule somewhere that says ugly people are ignorant and attractive people are intelligent. I had consistently been told that I was attractive, and I had been a good student in school. Now I began to question my own mental ability. Maybe my good grades related more to the way I had looked than the way I thought. Maybe my attractive body had been responsible for my graduating from college on the president's list. Maybe that is why I had been awarded academic scholarships and honors. Now that I was no longer physically attractive, I felt that I must no longer be intelligent. Ugly people do not deserve such honors and attention. But none of my physicians had ever explained that my physical illness had affected brain cells!

This lack of dignity crept in as I recognized how much knowledge is respected. To not know something means ignorance. Ignorance is not accepted or respected. Therefore, power is assigned to those who know. The more you know, the more power you must have.

So what could I say to the constant string of well-meaning persons who insisted on knowing something? My illness was laced with ambiguity. It simply lacked definition. Soon I realized that people were far more comfortable with facts than speculation. Many were immobilized by what they did not know. "Have they found out what's wrong with you yet?" was a common question. Because lack of information brought obvious uncomfortable feelings, people began to fill in the blanks to satisfy their own longing to know. To complicate matters, many versions began to erupt—rumors.

Until now, my tendency had been to deliberately choose not to learn more for fear of hurting more. Maybe I felt what I did not know would not hurt me. I came to realize that I stood alone. People were demanding to know. Friends could not tolerate ignorance and were determined to find out—even if the knowledge meant pain to me. My privacy was curtly invaded.

In the maze of uncertainties which surrounded this disease of unknown origin, it was most difficult to explain the diagnosis. I felt distance from some.

"If she is not going to get well, perhaps I should not get too involved." This was the attitude of a few well-meaning individuals.

My dignity was denied *emotionally*. I was elated at first with the number of people who responded to my pain. But soon I recognized that some of these well-meaning friends were enjoying my pain. The phone rang constantly with curious people who merely wanted to play a part in saving my life. Each had a secret remedy or advice: "Eat bananas, and drink eight glasses of water." Even more humiliating were those who insisted they knew exactly what I was going through. How could they? I was not sure that even I knew.

And then there were comments like: "How much do you weigh?" "I wish I could give you some of my fat!" "If they find out what you have, maybe I can catch it."

The mystery of my disease had puzzled medical professionals. I became a popular conversation topic at parties, professional medical meetings, many dinner tables, and even bar mitzvahs.

Humiliation hovered over my every action, it seemed. My every movement became a commentary on illness.

I continued to receive dozens of cards and letters almost daily. As I walked back to my condo from my mailbox one day, I was eager to get inside. I had received a small package. I realized that the sender had failed to indicate a return address. Not knowing who it was from made my excitement even greater. I enjoyed getting gifts. Quickly, I ripped through the brown paper and volumes of tape. It was a book. Carefully tucked between the pages was a note.

Dear Marsha:
You do not know me that well, but we are friends. I am writing this note to encourage you to get real help. I am also sending you this book because it helped me so much. It helped me find release from the same disease that I am confident is killing you. I know you think you are fooling the world with this "unknown" disease, but the truth is, you are just like me—anorexic. You know it! Admit it before it is too late. You will not get better until you do. I never got as bad as you, but I remember the prison in which I lived. I remember throwing up at least half a dozen times each day. I remember never finding a place where the guilt and the fear were not overwhelming. You are hiding, I think. I want God to free you. But you must go public. God can heal you. I hope you receive this message in love.

An anonymous friend!

I sank to the floor and began to feel faint. I simply was not able to conceive how anyone could really think that. Well, yes—maybe doctors who had to put something down or their reputations were on the line—but not a friend. Which "friend"? Would I have to live the rest of my life wondering who?

Not knowing who wrote the note became even more difficult to accept than the fact that someone thought I was anorexic. The list of "who" became wider and more inclusive. I suspected nearly everyone. I became unconsciously uncomfortable being around or even eating in front of almost everyone. After all, they might be wondering when and if I was going to throw up.

All around, people, I thought, were staring. No, it was not in my head. It was true. I had enjoyed attention in the past, but this was different. Even children looked frightened when they saw my 5'7", 84-pound body. I wanted to stay inside to protect myself from the arrows of accusation and humiliation. But somehow I realized that developing agoraphobia was a possibility for someone beginning to feel the whirlwind of paranoia. I exercised control by forcing myself to go to the grocery store, the mailbox, the library, my church, and a special sanctuary from the storm: McDonald's.

On another walk to my mailbox, I noticed two men on the roof of the condo building next to mine. They were speaking loudly, obviously intending to be heard.

"Hey, Bill. Look at that woman! Do you really think she feels she is turning us on? She makes me sick, just looking at her. I guess she thinks she's fat."

"Hey, baby, you're getting too fat!"

I could not believe I spoke back so boldly: "At least fat people can change. Being ugly is permanent."

I escaped into my condo. I wanted to scream and set the record straight. I wanted to run, but I didn't know where.

These types of encounters became the norm, rather than the unexpected.

In a plea for security, I realized that only our Father is security. I cannot identify my good with my body, or who I am with, what I do, or where I am. When those things change, and eventually they all do, I am forced to either shift my perspective or sink.

As I struggled to stay above the waves of humiliation, I began to realize that my good must go deeper than this physical cavity. It was only as I accepted myself did others accept me. But this acceptance was not always in the form in which I had received it before or by the same people.

Self-esteem began to creep back into my life once I realized that the only way to increase my self-worth was to identify myself with my Father. But it came not in the form of self-esteem but God-esteem. I began to see through different eyes —eyes of humility. I began to respect those who I once identified as ugly and ignorant. I realized their significance as members of the human race. They, too, were people of worth. They had feelings. They had value.

I had been so guilty in the past of passing judgment. Now I had been judged—unjustly. People who would be classified as rejects by most standards became my teachers. After all, they had been trying to overcome the stigma of rejection for many years. I began to learn from them as they became my friends.

My condo was small. I spent nearly twenty-four hours a day there. I began to crave other places in which to spend my time. I discovered that McDonald's opened at 6:00 AM. So I decided to join the white-collar breakfast bunch even though I no longer worked. Soon, I began to take my Bible and notebook to pull out after breakfast. It wasn't long until I was spending the entire morning, at least five days a week, at the golden arches.

After a few days, I noticed Sarah, who worked behind the

counter. She was not an attractive person physically. She was overweight. Her teeth were crooked, her complexion was scarred, her hair stringy, and she seemed sort of slow mentally. She never looked up when taking orders. One morning, I was determined to look her in the eyes and say good morning.

"Sarah, it is a great day!"

It worked. She looked up and smiled.

"How did you know my name? No one has ever called me by my name here," she said.

"Your name tag."

The next morning when I arrived, Sarah looked at me.

"Good morning. Coffee?"

"How did you remember, Sarah?" I asked.

"I watch you. Every day, you drink coffee and read. We all talk about you. Are you a famous writer or something? After all, you write for hours. We have all decided that maybe you are writing a book!"

"Oh, Sarah! A book—I could write a book. Maybe one day what I write in this white notebook will be a book."

I began to notice her. She spent all of her time, when not behind the counter, sweeping the floor in my area. I always sat in the same place—the corner next to the large front window. My corner was spotless.

"You certainly are a hard worker," I said one morning as her broom chased a straw wrapper across the already-shiny floor.

"I like things to look good. Say, Ramon—he's the Mexican guy who washes the windows—wanted me to ask you what you do. I mean, are you married? Do you have a job? He was afraid to ask you himself. He just thinks you are nice and pretty, and, well, you are."

"Sarah, you and Ramon are both nice."

Silently, I pondered the word *pretty*. That was the first time someone had said that in—well, I can't remember when.

"I have been writing in my journal about you. These are my private thoughts. I have been learning a lot lately. Maybe I am

taking a course in life management. Anyway, you and Ramon
are in my book.

"I have a job, but I am not working right now. You could say
I am taking a little vacation. Anyway, I just enjoy coming here.
I hope it is OK."

Sarah's eyes were fixed on the white notebook.

"I'd like to read it. No one has ever written anything about
me. What did you say?"

"Oh, I said that I noticed you and felt happy when we
learned each other's names the other day. I said I wanted to
learn from you."

"Learn from me? I didn't even finish high school. What can
you learn from me?"

"Well, Sarah, we will simply have to spend time together to
know that."

Sarah smiled. "I get breaks. I could take them in the morning
with you. Maybe we could talk?"

"Sarah! Would you? I would love that. Tomorrow?"

"Tomorrow."

It was now approaching 9:00. Usually I stayed later than
that, but I had to check in with Dr. Kennedy. I gathered my
pens, my copy of *My Utmost for His Highest* by Oswald Chambers, my notebook, and Bible and stuffed it all into my brief-
case. If I hurried, I could stop by the post office to mail the stack
of letters I had written that morning to friends. Oh, yes, writing friends helped with the loneliness.

On many days, I had to leave McDonald's not just because
of the appointment with Dr. Kennedy. Usually between 9:30
and 10:00, the fever ripped through my body. It was almost
unbearable at times. It was worse now, because I was determined to become drug free. So, I often left to escape to a
bathtub full of ice cubes.

I often confessed the pain to the Father. I had to get the
emotions out. Writing became one way to cope. I began to

learn that my ministry was not of brilliant moments but of walking in the light of ordinary days.

Early the following morning, I joined the ranks of the hungry working force. Rather than choosing the shorter line, I chose Sarah's. She was not the fastest on the cash register, but I was not exactly in a hurry. She spotted me.

Sarah looked different. Her hair was clean and combed neatly with an ornament holding it in place. Her uniform was ironed, and she had on makeup, even though it was uneven.

I leaned over the counter and whispered, "Do you have a date today?"

Sarah laughed. "Yeah, you!"

"You look terrific, Sarah."

"No, Marsha. You are the one who looks terrific."

I could hardly see that. I wore the same blue jogging suit every day. *What is beauty?* I thought. *Is it something we project? Is it physical?* I did know that Sarah was becoming more beautiful to me every day.

"I have a break at 7:30. Is that OK?"

"You bet. I will be waiting."

I handed Sarah two quarters for the coffee.

"No, it's on me today."

I simply smiled and accepted Sarah's simple gift of a cup of coffee. Thoughts of a coffee-cup ministry began to tickle my imagination.

The first visit seemed awkward for both of us. I simply asked questions. Sarah talked freely but never looked directly into my eyes.

She was from a poor family. She was very young, unmarried, and the mother of a fifteen-month-old girl. The more Sarah talked, the more I realized we had absolutely nothing in common.

Sarah had not completed high school. She was living with her mother but hoped soon to buy a mobile home. This would be the first major purchase of her life. She had spent her entire life in Irving, Texas—a bedroom community in the Dallas area. She had never traveled outside of a thirty-mile radius of her home.

How did my life-style compare to Sarah's? I had traveled in nearly every state and many foreign countries. I had three degrees and was hoping for a fourth, a doctorate in education. She was a mother. I was not. She knew nothing of Jesus; I was from a Christian background. She was 17; I was 30. Our body sizes were different. Our hobbies had nothing in common. She enjoyed spending free time watching TV; I enjoyed reading, writing, and creating. But what difference did it make? None! I had learned to celebrate the difference. What we had in common was far more than age, hobbies, and life-style. Our bond came from one thing. We were both hungry for acceptance and freedom from judgment. Sarah accepted me. I accepted Sarah. We were simply "one beggar trying to tell the other where to find bread."

I visited with Sarah nearly daily. Weeks and months passed. Ramon and the others began to dominate my thoughts. I now lived in two worlds. A world of pain and illness—that was the condo and medical center. Then there was a sanctuary from my storm—McDonald's. My habits soon became a positive addiction. I was addicted to the love and ability to see beyond myself. I saw needs far different than my own. My self-centered life began to take on a new focus. I began to identify a field that was unreaped. This field responded to what I had to give. Weak as I was physically, I was a strength to these new friends whom earlier I never would have noticed. I began to see a field outside my window.

How can God use me? I often thought. I am tired. I am sick. I am spent. How could God use someone like me in Sarah's and Ramon's lives? Then, I would remember. The power for ministry does not come from my strength. God is the source of power—the same as the "voice" in the wind. He used a loaf of bread to feed the thousands; surely He could use me to feed Sarah and Ramon.

My new friends did not know about my illness. I liked it that way. I enjoyed not being associated with illness. I enjoyed being able to talk about something besides myself. What I learned during those months were among the greatest lessons I had learned so far in my life. Sarah and Ramon taught me about real love, acceptance, and humility.

Because of them, I learned that I did not have to work in a Christian profession to have a personal ministry. My ministry did not need to be so tied to a place or job that I could not minister if I was not there. It was then that I was inducted into a small fraternity of those called to be "ragpickers."

I got the "ragpicking" idea from Og Mandino's book, *The Greatest Miracle in the World*. He describes an old man whose purpose in life was simply to be a "ragpicker." For those of us who had escaped the Depression, he explained that a "ragpicker" made it his or her occupation to search for wasted materials discarded by others.

In a brief interview with this "junk man," Mandino questioned why anyone would become a "ragpicker" by choice. These are trying days today but not days of depression. The elderly gentleman quietly suggested that he was not that kind of ragpicker. What he sought was much more valuable than cans or paper. He was searching for waste of the human kind— "people who have been discarded by others, or even themselves, people who still have great potential but have lost their self-esteem and their desire for a better life. When I find them I try to change their lives for the better, give them a new sense of hope and direction and help them return from their living death which to me is the 'greatest miracle in the world'" (Mandino).

Suddenly, I realized that being a ragpicker of the human variety was my kind of business.

But I decided that I must go one step further. I was convinced that I must not only be one who picks up those rejected by others but one who is willing to be picked up—allowing them the joy of being used to extend God's good to me. By denying anyone the opportunity to give to me, I denied God's love channeled through them. It meant not being selective about who could minister to me; it also meant not being selective about those to whom I ministered.

I soon learned what I received from others must be anointed with love, respect, and the willingness to learn from them. Therefore, everyone, everything, and anytime could become my teacher. I began to learn something awesome about myself when I realized that a dignity denied deepened my humility. By being willing to learn from those I had classified as lower than myself, those who had been rejected by others, I learned something marvelous about myself and my Father.

Sarah taught me about a life I had never known. I taught Sarah about a life she had never known. Together we gave each other a reason to live and fight. The love and compassion we shared was contagious. Soon the little fraternity of ragpickers spread to Ramon, Sandra, and Lori (the supervisor). Sarah became my reason for getting up in the morning and going to bed early and unsedated.

I began to pray for an opportunity to share my faith in Jesus Christ with her. It happened. I concluded by sharing that I never wanted to forget the winter. It was the winter that had taught me to live. I wondered if through my winter others could find life.

After sharing all the things I wanted my new friend to know about Jesus, a young woman nearer my age came to our booth. Her eyes were red. She looked as if she had been awake all night.

"Can I ask you a question?"

"Sit down, sure!"

"That stuff that you just told that woman." She looked at Sarah. "Will it work for me?"

"Of course! You must have overheard our conversation," I said.

The unnamed woman explained: "I have some problems. I came here to think. I had planned to go home to take my life—commit suicide. Can you help me?"

Sarah looked at me as if to say, *Help her, Marsha.*

"I am absolutely certain who can. He helped me when I felt I had no reason to live. I then shared my pilgrimage of the past year. Sarah's eyes were totally fixed on me. She hung onto every word. Even though we had spent months of mornings together, this was the first Sarah knew of my illness. "He can change your life, too. You choose."

Sarah's break was over. She excused herself and went back to work a very reflective young lady. Our new friend simply stared into space. "I must go now," she said.

I was horrified. I followed her to her car. She sat for minutes with her head heavy on the steering wheel.

"I care what happens to you."

"I think you do. Why?"

"Because He loved me first, I guess."

"Are you sure it will work for me?" she said.

"I am positive."

We prayed. She left. I ran inside and asked Sarah and Lori if I could use their phone. I called some friends to pray for this new friend. I never saw her again, but I feel confident that some day I will.

My new friends taught me about life and gave me a reason to continue my fight to live. They taught me to hope that I would never forget the winter or question it when it comes again. Had it not been for my winter and the dignity denied, I might never have been in a position to listen to the voice of humility that was now enhancing and embracing all of my life. Had it not been for the winter, there would never have been hope for spring.

Reflections of Acceptance

Running deep within each of us is a plea for acceptance. It is manifested in many ways. We crave acceptance, but we feel rejection.

Whether or not rejection is real is not significant to the one feeling rejected. The degree to which we feel rejected varies. And we deal with it by using various escapes. My escapes were sleeping, denial, narcotics and sedatives, and even serious thoughts of suicide. My need to escape came because of what happened to my body. But we are more than bodies; we are souls unlike any of God's other creations.

Real acceptance comes when body and soul learn to accept each other. That is internal acceptance which has eternal implications.

As we begin to accept ourselves completely, our lacks and limitations diminish, and our own magnificence increases. That is not self-consciousness. Rather, it is self-esteem rooted in God-esteem.

As I identify whose I am and my Kingdom heritage, my position in life is naturally elevated. After all, my Father created me and the universe. He also created all of the "Sarahs" in the world. To reject the "Sarahs" is to reject the Creator. To accept the "Sarahs" is to demonstrate an enormous level of God-esteem. I no longer have a need to judge, justify, or set the record straight when it comes to relationships. My job is simply to be a "ragpicker" of the human kind.

Such identity frees me to see through the eyes of humility— eyes that do not compare, eyes that simply focus on caring. There is no need to think about the way it used to be or could be—only the way it is. I can celebrate by using the wind from the storms.

Because we share the same Creator, no one is below us. Likewise, no one is above us. We are all created in His own image. Therefore, when we put down others, we are only putting down ourselves. It's a personal demotion. It is a symptom of a lack of our own God-esteem. It says that we have refused to recognize that the same Creator created all persons —you, them, and us.

To be willing to learn from others—regardless of the world's view of their positions in life—may well be the highest example of security, not to mention learning.

To be a "ragpicker" of the human kind emulates the lifestyle of Jesus Christ. He suffered rejection, but He loved and accepted in far greater proportion than His rejection. If He can accept those who falsely accused Him, those who beat Him, those who murdered Him, can I not choose to accept all persons? It is then, and only then, that I am exalted in humility.

It is truly springtime as I recognize the birth of my dignity in Christ.

Why does my heart feel faint
And my life a compromise?
When did my dreams turn into nightmares?
They have crumbled before my eyes.

I am stripped of all I am
Left only with foolish pride
I cannot stand on my own
I have no place to go
Where is my home?
Am I really just passing through?

I am tired, spent, weary
My destiny denied
I feel stripped and barren
Ashamed of who I am.

But, I will someday be freed
Of the pain that covers me
And the trials
They too will one day end
Until then
I will dwell in the shadows of Your wings.

"I AM who I AM," You say
"Willing to help, willing to heal
I will not deny you
I am willing to heal.

So, here I am, Father
Broken, humble, and bent
Ready for Your plan
Point me to another day
Celebrate Your life in me once more.

—Marsha Spradlin

11
Designing My Destiny

There is a time for everything,
and a season for every activity under heaven
(Eccl. 3:1).

"What time is it?" In a panic, I grabbed my glasses off the table next to the bed and strained to read the clock on the wall. It wasn't there. The clock was gone! I had watched the hands slowly revolve hour after hour. Where is the clock? Soon, I was awake enough to realize that it was only a dream. For a fleeting moment, I thought I was back in ICU. I was relieved!

I had experienced this dream several times since being released from the hospital nearly four months earlier. The trauma of the ICU experience had apparently made a deeper impression on my subconscious than I had realized.

Each dream was the same. I would suddenly awaken in the night desperately looking for the clock. If it was still there, I decided I must still be alive. But I knew that if the clock were gone, I had died. It was dreadful.

Usually, once awake, I could not return to sleep easily, so I would simply get up early. Each day started the same way, enveloped with questions. Why get up anyway? What is the real point of trying so hard to stay alive? I continued to starve for answers about the reason I had survived so far. As I searched, I desperately fought to hang on to any sign of progress. It almost did not exist. I continued to stay much the same. Recovery was not obvious to me or Dr. Kennedy.

If it had not been for Sarah and Ramon, I probably could not have faced each day. They continued to give me courage. With the exception of my "sanctuary under the arches," frequent visits to the medical center were the only consistency in my life. With each visit, I was stuck, pricked, poked, questioned, and given no real hope.

Since I was the most consistent part of Dr. Kennedy's practice, I had been assigned my very own examination room. Why not? I spent almost as much time there as I did at home. Dr. Kennedy even decorated it with one of my favorite Scripture verses.

My days were routine. Each visit to the medical center ended with a long distance call to Mother.

"Eighty-four and a half today, Mother. White blood count is down (or up a fraction). No real change. I'll call the day after tomorrow. Love ya!"

The drive home was usually depressing. I had to go within one block of my office. I would always notice that life was going on without me. Staff members were still loading cars with conference materials, catching airplanes, and traveling all over Texas with a purpose. Not me. I simply drove home, holding my right hand which was usually throbbing with pain from the complications of the many blood tests and a set of bad veins. The veins had now built enormous scar tissue. Even getting a blood sample was an ordeal. In addition to the throbbing, I was still plagued with the midmorning fever.

If I hurry, I can get home and out of the heat before it elevates too high. Because of the fever, I spent most of the afternoon asleep only to wake up at supper time feeling lonely and guilty for not having accomplished anything significant. I had no real purpose for my day.

"How can I sleep all afternoon when I have been given a second chance to be awake and alive?" I asked myself. I felt deeply that my life had been given back to me. Even so, I became overwhelmed with the guilt of not knowing how to make my days meaningful. Perhaps the frequent nightmares of the clock made this point obvious. I still could not escape my illness. If only I could make time or even illness my friend, I might have a chance to figure out what to do with the remaining fragments of my life.

I no longer felt that time was a luxury. I wanted badly to capture each moment and embrace it tightly. I became preoccupied with time. I felt the need to capitalize on each moment. Perhaps it was the fear of the unknown or even the fear that I would not wisely use the days that had been given back to me. Regardless, time was fleeting, and I could not get a handle on it. I felt the urgency to live quickly. After all, time was running out.

Where was this life that had been given back to me? Just as sand slipped through the hour glass of time, my days slipped through my own life without direction and purpose. If only I could find out where it is going! If I could simply grasp it, embrace it, hold it, touch it, catch it, or stop it. Regardless of how hard I tried, the hours continued to slip through meaningless days. Could time ever become my friend? Could it ever bring me the joy of the new day and the hope that deepens as the day lets go into night?

Time was a mystery. In some ways, it was a greater mystery than my own illness. Are the most beautiful experiences in life always mysteries?

Questions about this mystery dominated my thoughts. Does time belong to me? If so, how should I spend it? Could I ever give back the days that had been given back to me? Who answers these questions, anyway?

I was a "type A" personality. "Type A" stays busy. I prefer the word *industrious.* When there is nothing pressing to do, we create something. The mandate from my good physician was rest, rest, rest. Do nothing but rest. A "type A" sometimes interprets rest as laziness. Therefore, rest or lack of activity causes stress.

Dr. Kennedy began to see my positive spirit deteriorate. I became ambivalent.

"What you need is a little vacation. You have been out of the hospital now about four months, and you have not been outside the city limits. How does a trip to Mobile sound?"

"You mean it? I can drive home?"

"Who said anything about driving? No way. You can fly home for a couple of days. The change would be good. But don't forget to come back. A couple of days is about as long as we can go around here without your 10:00 check-in."

I raced to the elevator and punched P. The telephones were in the plaza. There I called Mom.

"Can you stand me again, for a weekend? Dr. Kennedy thinks I am strong enough for the trip, if I fly. Of course, I have to get a blue suitcase for all of the antibiotics. He said he would give me the name of a doctor in Mobile we could call if I got into trouble."

Early Friday morning, Barbara loaded the car with my three suitcases for the two-day trip. I felt like a kid going away to summer camp. I could hardly wait. Yet, in the midst of the excitement, I feared leaving Dallas—my doctor, my hospital, my charts.

Daddy met my plane. As we embraced, we each remembered our last good-bye. I could still see him looking up from the parking lot to the window of room 6435 at the medical center. Even at that distance, we could feel each other's love and see each other's tears. This was a special moment. We never knew I would ever come home again.

The drive to our house was quiet.

"Dad, where's Mom?" I knew something was up. She was probably home cooking my favorite lunch: chicken, baked potatoes, and squash casserole.

"Your mom's not feeling too good, honey. We think it's a kidney stone. I took her to the doctor, and he is trying to wash it out of her. I have decided that we are both better patients than your mother."

Arriving home was special. Dad put my suitcases in my old room. Even though Mother now called my room the "guest room," it was still "my" room as far as I was concerned. In it were my pictures, my telephone, my furniture, and my memories of earlier days. Next to my bed was Mama Amy's picture and the Bible I had given her when I was in the eighth grade. I missed her most often when I was home. For more than eighteen years, she had been my roommate.

Mother was certainly not running races, but she did not appear to be in terrific pain. We spent most of the afternoon sitting out on the patio. I enjoyed going through boxes of high school memorabilia. I found my old yearbooks and read the messages of hundreds of high school friends scribbled throughout. Most lacked originality: "Marsha, you're a cute girl. You should go far in life!" Ah, ha! There it is again. You will make it in life if you're cute. Oh, well. I still loved those friends who had been so special to me over a decade ago. Mother knew that. She also knew I wanted privacy during this trip. No one knew I was in Mobile, except Larry and Teresa.

Late Friday night, Daddy rushed into my bedroom. "Honey, get your shoes on. I am taking your mom to the hospital. She is in terrific pain. We need to hurry."

And hurry we did. As we pulled up to the emergency room, a nurse and an attendant with a wheelchair met us. Quickly, yet carefully, they moved Mother from the car to the chair. "Marsha, you get her settled while I park the car."

The nurses noticed her obvious pain. Rather than filling out the volumes of papers first, they took Mother directly into an examination room. I was reluctant to enter the treatment area. But Mother's nurse signaled for me to follow, and I did.

I was completely focused on Mother and her pain. Yet, an unidentified feeling rushed in. I was unable to stop it or control it. There were too many memories: beeps, green curtains, monitors, computer terminals, bright lights, white sheets, stainless steel, and a large clock on the wall. Suddenly, I felt faint. The sounds became echoes in the distance. A burning sensation covered my body. I felt the ringing of utter terror inside. My skin turned completely white. In spite of her pain, Mother knew what was happening. She grabbed my arm and shouted, "Get out of here. Please, get her out of here, quick!"

I felt myself sinking. With my head tucked near my stomach, I ran toward double doors—totally disoriented. I escaped through the hallway and exited through the first door I opened. It led to a stairwell. I leaned against the cold, dirty concrete wall. Slowly, I sank to the floor and curled into a tight position. I braced my arms around myself trying to stop shivering. Silently, I cried, "No! Please don't let me die, again. Not in there."

I must have sat in the stairwell over an hour. Once the tears began to flow, I knew I would be OK. I cried like never before. Once I regained my composure, I knew the trauma was not happening to me. But for a moment, I felt the total impact of the entire ICU experience directing a solid blow to my emotions. The terror became even more intense as I associated my pain with Mother. Could it happen to her?

Daddy had been searching the entire hospital for over an hour. When he found me, nothing can describe the comfort as he gently explained what I mentally knew to be true, but my emotions had simply refused to accept.

"You've got to face it sometime, honey. You didn't die. You are not to blame for your pain or for the pain we have all been through. You are not a victim of the world you see. Your mother is being helped. She is not dying. You must go back in there."

"Not now, Daddy."

"If not now, when?"

I felt like a bird with a broken wing locked inside a tiny cage. Just as my own daddy talked to me, I heard my Heavenly

Father cry out: "My greatest desire is to set you free. But every time I try to touch you, you flap your wings wildly to fly away. Your pain has taken away your sight. Your agony will only grow as you continue this mindless flight. And you still think I'm the cause of all this. Oh, Marsha, you remind Me of a frightened child. You say you want to trust Me, but you watch fearfully from afar. I already hold everything you long for right in My hand. I am waiting for you to take My hand in yours. My love will be salve for your wounds and will elevate you above the storm, so you won't need to be afraid. All you have to do is come to Me."

Daddy spoke again, "Marsha, honey, are you coming?" The frightened child in me reached for his hand. Slowly and totally exhausted from the emotional agony of the experience, I dug deep for courage. As I took my daddy's hand, I took my Father's hand. As I entered my dungeon, I faced my fears once again. As I saw Mother's pain relieved, I was freed from my own prison of fear. Yes, the key to my prison cell had been firmly tucked inside myself all along!

I returned to Dallas on Sunday. As my plane landed, my spirit soared above the clouds. Barbara greeted me with a hug and a warm smile. Immediately, she recognized a difference.

What was different?

I had peace. I had trust. I felt the security of the Father who had chosen me. I had a real sense of purpose instead of a need to control the minutes of the day. I had a vision of hope instead of despair. I felt relaxed instead of intense in not wanting to waste a minute. I was content to wait patiently to understand why I had survived when Karen had not.

Early Monday morning, I walked to my mirror and announced, "It's a great day, and I feel great." I really did not, but compared to the emotional prison I had experienced, I did feel relief.

With this in my mind, I stuffed my Bible, Oswald Chambers's devotional book, and my white notebook into my brief-case and headed toward my "sanctuary." Sarah had been wondering where I had slipped off to. My table was clean and waiting for me. I spread out my Bible, opened my notebook, and breathed in God's Word for me:

Dear Father:
    I have just read Psalm 139! Why have I been so uptight? I guess I felt I was the only one who could be trusted. I hereby authorize You to take control of my life and my time. After all, You designed my every part. You said You would never leave me nor forsake me. You have been here all along. Why have I not noticed?
    I'm looking at my hands. Even though they're a little scarred, they're magnificent. They are unique and wonderful. Now I'm considering my eyes. Do they really contain countless receptors that allow me to see the snow falling and the seasons changing? And You made my ears. I can hear Sarah and Ramon laughing. I'm so glad my ears have picked up the sounds of rolling thunder, the wind blowing through the trees, and the words *I love you!* I have working vocal chords. Does any other creature have anything comparable to the human voice? My body may be small, but You made it complete. You did not make me rigid like a tree. No, You gave me a body that can move quickly. As I do, I can touch others in love. Someone told me that you synchronize 500 muscles, 200 bones, and 700 miles of nerves. Is that true?
    There is no one like me. I am like a snowflake. I am rare. I must have purpose for the time You have given me. I must give myself away.
    Yes, Father, I will give my rarity away. I will strive not to walk as my brother or talk as my leader but to be myself. I shall not conform any longer to the patterns of the world, but I will seek to be transformed. That's it.
    You have transformed me by renewing my mind. I have been *transformed one winter!* Whatever happens, regardless of the days ahead, may I never forget the winter.

You have searched me. You know me. There is none other like me. I am wonderfully made. Yes, a snowflake!

Father, I am hearing You say, "I have no body now but you." Take me, Father. For I am completely Yours. As You take me, design my days to be filled with purpose, meaning, and life. My time is Your time. Your time is my life. I have recognized that I was born into Your arms. You are still my refuge. From my first breath, You have always been my security. You have been my shelter. As my days go by before Your eyes like the days rushing into night, I will not let the pressure of time steal my dream. Instead, I will let time give me hope.

I have chosen to follow You. You have freed me from my cage. You are the beginning and the end. Who am I to control my days? May my every thought be from You. May my every breath adore You. May my every move exalt Your holy name. You are my reason for living. I have no other purpose.

I know now that my fear of dying was not fear of dying at all, but the sorrow of never having lived with a purpose. I can die now. I have a purpose! I hear it loudly ringing like church bells on Christmas morning. But what is even clearer and ringing even louder is the message that I am free to live. I am no longer on trial for a crime I did not commit. So, if it's OK with You, can we live together here a little longer? You decide. Meanwhile, let my life be a signature of Your love.

Joyfully,

MARSHA

The design of my days took a different form. Security and solitude were very present. Days were still rushing into the night. But the nights were no longer darkened with doubts. No longer did I feel the need to sleep with my door unlocked.

I noticed very little change at first, but, little by little, my life began to take shape. As I spent hours with my Teacher each day, my mind was renewed and my life transformed.

I began each day by asking the Father to organize my day and set my priorities. As I spent time with Him daily at my "sanctuary" under the golden arches, purpose became obviously twofold: God and people. I began to recognize that I was created to have fellowship with the Creator and fellowship with His creation. My purpose involved relationship—with my Father and with my brothers and sisters.

Soon I realized that when I chose to grasp time and hold on to it for myself, I lost it. Only when I used time as it was designed to be used did I make a permanent investment that multiplied and yielded precious eternal dividends.

As He designed my days, I met myself. Up until then, I needed to control the design of my daily activities. I did not know what I needed or who needed me. But He did. Each day became a new experience and an adventure into the mysteries of time.

Each day also brought new opportunities to say thank you for the gift of life. As He designed my days, He designed not only my destiny but the destinies of others. He taught me to let go of fruitless time consumers in my life to make room for things and people I did need or who needed me. It's called balance. The balance included spiritual, social, mental, emotional, and physical. As I participated in His plan for my total recovery, I kept detailed notes in my white journal. As I met Him daily to start my day, I always asked five basic questions:
1. What do I need to know today?
2. Where do I need to go today?
3. Who do I need to see today?
4. Why am I still alive today?
5. How do I look to You today, Father?

During the following months, I began to recognize time as my friend. My body began to slowly regain its form and energy. Likewise, my life regained its purpose.

Spiritually, I could not find enough time to be with the Father. I became addicted to His presence and to time spent in His Word. For hours and hours, I would read, underline, and write in my white notebook. Spiritual nuggets that had always been there seemed to fall into my head, heart, and soul. The joys were new every morning.

The fear of sharing my faith was gone. I did not find myself having to go out and look for people who needed to know God's good news. They were everywhere. Often they came to me. Over and over, Sarah and I spent her breaks sharing Christ with someone who walked into our "sanctuary under the arches." Ramon even wanted to know why Sarah was so different.

Physically, I began to feel stronger. I started walking twice a day—first only a half mile, then one and then two. I kept a close record of how many calories I burned in order to replenish all I spent. I continued doing isometrics and even lifted one-pound weights to strengthen my arms.

Socially, relationships became top priority. The more time I gave away, the more time I seemed to have available. I had little time to think about myself. I found new ways to say "I love you." I learned to cook and enjoyed entertaining a house full of friends. This meant buying groceries—often. I developed another Sarah-type relationship with Abbie at the grocery store.

Then, there was Hank, the tailor. He made enough money altering and then selling my clothes to send his daughter to college. I disposed of them because I knew I had to get rid of the things that were no longer a part of my life to make room for new things that were being introduced. Hank asked, "Why are you so happy when you look so sick?"

"Hank, do you know that God saved my life? Come on, wouldn't you smile?"

I didn't need more friendships. I simply needed to learn to be a friend to the friends I had. Hundreds had sent cards. It was time to get my act together and express a little love back to them. So, one by one, I personally wrote each person who had called or sent a card and each church that expressed concern. I counted nearly two thousand. That meant another new relationship with Ralph, the cashier at the post office who sold me rolls of stamps each week. He asked, "Why are you writing so many letters?"

"Wouldn't you, Ralph, if you thought people's prayers had saved your life?"

Mental alertness became important. I sought ways to keep my brain in good working order. Because Barbara was still traveling and trying to keep her office running full steam, I managed to sneak a project or two from her "to-do" stack just to stay in shape. I did not intend on staying out of professional commission forever, but I had come to realize that my happiness and ministry were not linked to my old job.

Mental fitness also included the library. I got a library card. Each day after leaving Sarah and Ramon, I would stop by the library for more books on how to become the person God wanted me to be. I read a book a day. I met Becky, the librarian who likewise wondered why I was her most consistent customer. Becky was another story of love.

Emotionally, all was well. I fell in love with myself. Before, I would have thought that to be self-centered. But I now saw myself through different eyes. I needed to love myself. By doing so, I said to my Father, I love You because You made me wonderfully. That's called God-esteem! I simply enjoyed my solitude and my time alone with my Father. Each night, I would lie in bed and listen to Christian cassette tapes. The beautiful music imprinted my thoughts and emotions with a sort of spiritual therapy. I would go to sleep each night with the sweet messages of His love deeply impressed on my heart and mind. By sleeping with His messages of love planted firmly within, I felt the joy of being greeted each morning by my Father who simply kissed my life with His love.

My every need was cared for. Everything I ever longed for was within my reach. He had just been waiting for me to come to Him with arms outstretched.

Reflections on Purpose

Time is a mystery. Every great thought or action that has ever occurred has done so in time. The earth was created in time. It was in time that my inward parts were formed. Until now, I had not had time to think about it.

Most of my life had been jam packed. My list of things to do each day was usually running over. No, the list was not running over; I was. The tyranny of the urgent began to nibble at my day, bit by bit. My life had become one trivial pursuit. I finally realized I had not allowed *breathing* room, much less *being* room.

I remember my struggle in ICU to see out the tightly locked window that was too high to reach. I somehow thought if I could only look outside, I could capture the day. Or if only I could stop the hands on the clock. Ah, today is not confined to a clock, nor is it wrapped between the pages of a book. Today cannot even be found in a calendar.

Now is the only time there is. You see, today is decidedly different from any day that has ever been. I only get one chance to spend it. I can never go back and retrieve it. Most of us either live in yesterday or we are busily working on tomorrow's agenda.

There is value in the past. But it is very different from the present. The past, after all, brought us to today. There is value in tomorrow, but it lies only in a dream.

Where do time and purpose merge? I have come to believe that it is at the point of relationships—God's love relationships. Love is meaningful only as it is wrapped in the *now*. Love can only be expressed freely *now*. Like its friend Time, it cannot be captured or held. Like time, it can be found in everyone and everything in varying degrees. Like time, love patiently waits. But it waits actively, not passively. It continually offers itself in mutual revelation and mutual sharing. In love, *now* is the only time there is. It is neither lost in yesterday, nor does it crave tomorrow. Like time itself, love knows no age.

As we are freed from the preoccupation of thinking about the future, or even the past, we are freed to live today and love today. We allow the power of the love of God to heal our fears and make us all we can be in time. In time, we learn to imitate Christ whose love is not limited to time. Through love, I can live forever!

As I identify my purpose for living as loving God and loving others, my life has direction. Without it, I am unable to invest my time; I only abuse it. By knowing where I am going, I can know when I get there!

What are the opportunities for today? Today is interesting because within it, God has sheathed all of the good and perfect gifts that He wishes to give. By recognizing the gifts of today, we must recognize Him. Recognition is our choice. We likewise choose how to spend the gift of today. We can use it or lose it. We are the only ones who can make these decisions. To have time, we simply must live time. To have life, we simply must give ourselves and time away. This is where time and purpose merge. Only relationships with God and others capture the mystery of time. In love, we can feel the hands of time standing still. Love has eternal implications!

To increase my time, I must give my time away. I do that as I give a cup of water away in His name. I do that as I receive a cup of coffee from Sarah.

What is this amber glow that warms my soul?
I can't take it lightly
For it has torn down the walls of selfish pride
It has mended the broken spirit and lost desires

Your love has conquered my fears,
Your love has dried the stream of tears
Your love has added days to my life—golden years

So, I commit all my love to You
I could search the world over
And never find a single thing new;
You loved me then
You love me now
I commit my love to You

—MARSHA SPRADLIN

12
Effects of the Son

He will make your righteousness shine like the dawn,
the justice of your cause like the noonday sun.
(Ps. 37:6).

July 1984

The sun had risen. Painted clearly across the sky were brilliant shades of pink, blue, and purple. Accenting the colors was the reflection of the sun shimmering off the ocean. The familiar echoes of the waves escaping the ocean and clapping the sandy beach reminded me of a time that seemed long ago. Once again, I let the salty air breathe for me. I embraced the moment. This day was special. I wanted only to celebrate.

It was Fourth of July weekend. Mother and Daddy had planned their traditional family day at Gulf Shores. They were thrilled that Barbara could take a couple of days off to join our family.

Dr. Kennedy had agreed to let me go back home if Barbara would drive. So my friend and I embraced the weekend that marked the anniversary of my year of agony. We knew that this trip could trigger some painful memories for both of us. But we also knew it would be a celebration of a transformed life.

It was wonderful to be with Barbara and my family, but I wanted some time to myself. Early on the first morning at Gulf Shores, I slipped away. Exactly one year earlier, I had run on this beach. While its beauty was just as I had remembered, one thing was decidedly different—me. I was physically only a shadow of what I had been a year ago. So much had happened that could have left my body and soul battered, bruised, and abused. But while my body was weaker, my spirit made up the difference. It was stronger than ever before. I remembered 1 John 4:4: "The one who is in you is greater than the one who is in the world."

I knew my time alone on the beach was limited. It would not be long until it would be filled with people, beach balls, and the smell of hamburgers and hot dogs cooking over hot coals. But, at that moment, there were only two of us there, the Father and me.

I built my sanctuary under the sun by carefully spreading my blanket near the water. I unpacked my Bible, my white notebook, and *My Utmost for His Highest.* What a special place to start this special day! After only a moment, I felt frustrated. The gentle breeze was just strong enough to tangle the pages of my Bible. I fought it, then finally I gathered my books and pens and simply sat.

Over the next few moments, I experienced something entirely new. I could learn from the Father by simply listening and watching. While sitting on the cold sand, I learned a deeper meaning of love and divine security.

Quietly, I watched in amusement as the white foamy waves washed to shore and then quickly escaped to rejoin the ocean. They left behind a form of life, tiny sea crabs. They seemed stranded and almost frightened. Their little legs hurried them back toward the ocean as if their lives depended on it. The moment they reached the ocean, they were washed back to shore by another wave of liquid motion. The cycle repeated itself.

"Those silly sea crabs. If they would relax and simply be still, a stronger wave would take them back to the ocean where they belong. But no. They do not seem to see beyond this frightening moment."

Suddenly, I felt like a tiny sea crab. How could I have been so blind? Why had I been fighting it so long? The past year's experience felt like a mighty wave tossing me to and fro and even slapping me down at times. Just as I felt I was making progress and regaining strength, I felt knocked back into the storm. If only I could learn to rest, wait, and let God love me. Healing comes in waiting for the waves of pain to reverse their flow. It reverses when I simply acknowledge the presence of His love.

The rhythmic clapping of the waves brought a tranquil effect. I closed my eyes and chose to listen to the waves. But instead of hearing them reject the tiny crabs, I began to hear them rescuing them. This paralleled so beautifully my own spiritual healing. My Father had not brought me pain. But He had allowed it. He had not abandoned me. Instead, He stood ready to receive me and my pain.

I closed my eyes to pray. The sounds were so soothing. I felt sleepy. My mind began to gently float over the events of the past year. I considered how I could have reacted differently. I remembered the little crab. Just as it ran and panicked, I, too, had run as hard as I could from what seemed to be sabotaging me. Each time He spoke my name, I fled and the agonies accompanying my flight grew to be more than I could bear. I kept thinking He was making me feel this way. But I was the one who continued to dash myself against the stones when His love could have healed my wounds. I wanted to trust, but I only watched fearfully. Like a frightened child, I ran away at every move. Everything I had ever longed for was here waiting for me. Softly my heart heard Him speak. The message was not in words my ears could hear. Instead, it was a message of love that only my heart could understand:

> Marsha, wait! I am Love! To know Me is to know Love. My love is radically different from any love you have ever known. Come, come, to the water. Let Me love you!

I will love you, not because of who you are. My love does not depend on you. I am Love regardless.

I pledge not to love you because of what you do, because if you no longer do what you do, then I am not Love.

I cannot love you because of where you are, because if you leave where you are, then that would mean I am not Love.

My love for you does not depend on who you are, what you do, or even where you are. I love you because of who I am. I am Love.

Come. Let Me give you My gift of Love.

As the tide moved away from its shore, I felt Him gently placing a gift in my hands. It was simply love! With a desperate heart to know Him and with a courage to share Him, I accepted His gift. Only then, did I fully know who I was—I am an extension of love.

As I took the gift, I felt myself wrapped in it. Accepting His love was the wisest thing I had ever done.

I spent the entire morning sitting on the beach. Soon other people gathered, but it was OK. I still felt all alone in my sanctuary under the Son.

As the sun rose and began to warm my body and heal my outward parts, I felt the Son rising within my spirit, warming and healing my soul with His love. It deeply penetrated my wounds.

It was then that it happened. I felt healed in my soul. His love was so radically different from any I had ever known.

What did He teach me about love? I remembered the love chapter from 1 Corinthians 13. I heard Him tell me:

Marsha, if you speak in tongues of men and angels, but have not love, you are only a clanging cymbal. If you have the gift of prophecy, and if you can describe all of the mysteries and all knowledge, and if you have the faith to move mountains, but have not love, you are nothing. Love is patient, it is kind. It does not envy, it does not boast. It is not proud. It is not rude; it is not self-seeking. It is not easily angered; it does not record wrong. Oh, love does not delight in evil, but it rejoices with the truth. It always protects, it always trusts, it always hopes, it always preserves. Never, never will love fail. Marsha, there remains faith, hope, and love. But the greatest is *love* (adapted).

"Yes, Father, the greatest thing is love. And like time, in order to make more room for love, I must get rid of all the things within me that are unloving," I prayed.

As I breathed in the salty air, I breathed in His love. As I exhaled, I imagined exhaling the pain and bitterness as well as the anger that I still harbored against Jeff, Dr. Gonzales, the unknown person who sent the book, the two men on the roof, and others who had falsely accused me.

As I forgave each one, I made room for love. I loved Jeff, Dr. Gonzales, the unknown person, and the men on the roof. I began to view them with different eyes. They were not trying to capture me and rip me of my dignity. No, they, like myself, were only human beings searching for love.

I breathed in love for Jeff. "My sweet friend. You did not mean to complicate our lives so. If only you had known that you could find love in the Source of love. If I could face you now, I would give you not only my forgiveness, but I would point you toward a Source of love that we never shared."

I breathed in love for Dr. Gonzales. "You saved my life. It was you who noticed that my blood pressure was twenty points below what was being registered. If it had not been for you, I would not have been in ICU. If I had not been in ICU, I would not have known Debbie or had a chance to witness to Pam. Dear Dr. Gonzales, you loved me in your own way. You were so afraid that I would die. You did not know how to tell me how much you cared. I only wish I could tell you now how much I love you."

I breathed in love for my unknown friend. "Your life must have known pain far greater than my own. Whoever you are, you cared enough to risk. Thank you for loving me. Even though we did not share the same disease, we shared the pain. I wish to embrace you and encourage you with love from my Father. As your life is filled with His love, you will find the completeness and security that you are starving for."

I breathed in love for the two men working on the roof. "You must have been frightened. You felt helpless as you saw my emaciated body. May you come to know Him who is greater than he who is in the world. And by the way, I now believe ugly people can change!"

One by one, I breathed in love and forgiveness and breathed out the painful memories. The moments became hours. My soul became so full I simply had to stop. I knew I had to go and spend His love. I had realized that only by giving love away would I acknowledge I had received it. I could not give away what I did not have.

The beach became the secret place inside my heart to go in times of pain. Everywhere I went, I took my secret hiding place. Just as the seasons in my soul come and go, this one place would never change. It was peace that passes understanding. It was a blessing that would never fade. I prayed:

> Father, in our times alone, I have come to know the quiet words of Your love. They have gently changed my heart. Even in the storm, I am safe and warm in this secret hiding place inside my heart. You have covered me with grace. Here, I am peace. Here, I can stand while others may fall. Meet me here again.

The effects of the Son were obvious. Not only did others notice the change in my skin color but the change in the color of my soul as well.

The weekend was a celebration. As Barbara and I said good-bye to my family, we felt an unusual bonding. Like metal alloy, we felt united in the strongest way. We shared a common bond that nothing could destroy. Distance would separate us but never would space be between us. We could not be pulled apart for love bonded us together in the tightest way. It was the holy fusion that caused us to once again let go and say good-bye.

As we drove west, things were different from a year ago. We tried to listen to tapes. Each one brought tears of joy—especially "Leaning on the Everlasting Arms."

We had been driving for a couple of hours when suddenly I noticed it.

"Barbara, it's gone! It's gone!"

Barbara glanced into the back seat to try to identify what we had left in Mobile.

"No, the fever! The pain! I don't hurt. It's 10:30 AM. I always have fever at 10:30. I always hurt at 10:30. It's gone!"

Barbara pulled her car off the interstate and calmly put it in park. She took my hand and, with tears streaming down her face, said, "I know! I have known this time would come. I just didn't know it would be today. Marsh, God has done it! You have got to know that."

"We have to thank Him, Barb. Right now!"

There on the freeway, somewhere near Vicksburg, Mississippi, we bowed our heads in thanksgiving as we built an altar of praise and adoration. Instantly, I felt the attacks from the opponent.

"But Barb, what if it is just today? What if tomorrow it is back?"

"So what? That does not lessen the miracle of today."

It didn't lessen the miracle of the day or the days to come. I wish I could say the fever never returned again, but it did, but not as often and never for as long. Just as it slowly crept into my body, like a defeated dragon, it slowly limped away.

Monday, at 10:30 AM, I greeted Dr. Kennedy for my one hundredth visit that year. It was a celebration, not because of my centennial visit but because of the changes he noticed.

"Progress. I have never seen such slow progress, but it's here. Your weight is ninety pounds, and you are gaining about eight ounces a week. Your white blood count is still terrible, but who's counting? Not me. I gave up on you months ago. I decided if you were going to make it, it was because of a Greater Physician than I. How would you like to go back to work? Wait—before you get too excited—this is not a permanent arrangement. Just a couple days a week for maybe half a day? I talked with Joy last week. She wants you back, Marsha. She is willing to work with me."

"Yes, yes! When?"

"Let's try next week. Tuesday and Thursday. Just half a day at first. You will still see me on Monday, Wednesday, and Friday."

I kissed Dr. Kennedy on the cheek and raced to the elevator and punched P. I didn't know who to call first, Mother or Barbara. It didn't matter, really. I simply had to share my news. I was absolutely elated. As I left the hospital, I told everybody, even the parking lot attendant. Why not? They had all become my friends, so they rejoiced with me.

Driving home I made a slight detour to pass my office. I looked at my window. I could barely see it. Inside the window hung a two-by-four-foot stained-glass window—a beautiful flower with a butterfly. A single word was embossed in brilliant yellow—*Chosen!*

I suddenly felt confused. I was chosen, but for whom? I began to experience an identity crisis. I had sudden thoughts of Sarah and Ramon. Who will be there for them? Who will love them?

"You have chosen me to love these people who are considered rejects by others. How will I ever tell Sarah and Ramon? How will they ever understand?"

Tuesday morning, I entered my "sanctuary." I was greeted by Lori, Sarah's supervisor.

"Marsha! We got a letter today from headquarters. Someone has been writing to the top brass about us. We get letters from time to time from our general office but never one like this.

Someone wrote the president of the corporation and told them about Sarah and Ramon. Anyway, they are both getting promotions! The letter said the sender wished to remain anonymous. We know who did it. Thanks, Marsha. We have an award for you, our most outstanding customer."

Sarah, Ramon, Lori, and the rest of the breakfast bunch had put together an award out of McMuffin containers. I was also given a plastic coffee mug for free refills—forever.

Tears streamed down my face. Sure, I was thrilled about the love they were giving. But the tears were for reasons I could not express. I was afraid that in one week my coffee-cup ministry would be forever over. While I waited for Sarah to join me, I sought a word from the Father:

> Dear Father:
>
> Why do I feel this weakness in my soul? I should feel victorious. Next week, I go back to work as I take my first step toward a normal life. But, Father, my life can never be normal again. How can it after all that has happened? My vision is different. My mind has been transformed. What used to be important isn't anymore. I don't care about things that should make me successful by human standards. All I care about is never forgetting the winter. I am so afraid I will forget the winter after going back to work. Please, Father, only I know how You have transformed my mind and life. Let me never forget the winter.
>
> I don't want to stop up my ears to avoid hearing the faint cries of the poor man's child going by. If I do, I believe You that one day someone will turn a deaf ear to my cries. You do not want hope to die. You have asked me to become Your hands. Lord, I hurt with them. Their pain fills my eyes.
>
> "Then I heard the voice of the Lord saying, 'Whom shall I send, and who will go for Us?' Then I said, 'Here am I. Send me!' " (Isa. 6:8, NASB).
>
> I will go where the need is greater, if You will go before me, Father. But let me go with a humble spirit. Let my spirit be Your Spirit. May all who see me see the effects of the Son!

The week was one of both psychological and spiritual preparation. I thought leaving the hospital was a step in faith into the dark, but now I felt that going back to work was the greatest step in faith so far. It would be a testing ground for me. Would I continue to grow and minister when life was normal? Ah, what is normal?

Barbara continued to be sensitive. On Saturday morning, we took a trial run from home to work. We got up, had breakfast, dressed, and were in the car by 8:00.

"No one will be at the building, Marsha. This will give you a chance to at least lay eyes on your desk before your first official day back. Let's take some of your plants. Your office needs a little life."

We arrived downtown at 8:20. I had not been inside the doors of our office building for nearly nine months. Strange feelings of both grief and joy flooded my emotions. We stepped on the elevator. I instantly punched ten.

"Marsh, where are we going?"

"To our office."

"Oh, Marsha, don't you remember? We are on the eleventh floor."

Tears ripped through my composure. "Barbara, Dr. Kennedy's office is on the tenth floor. It is the only place I have been this year. I can't remember what my office even looks like. But I can describe in detail my examination room. Barb, I don't think I can do it. I can never go back. It will never be the same here."

Barbara reached out and wrapped her arms around my shoulder and tightly squeezed.

"Marsh, let go. You have to let go. God's timing is perfect. You have got to trust Him."

"But, Barb, I don't even remember where my files are. I am not even sure what I do here. It will take months to dig out. Maybe I should quit."

"You are not a quitter. You are a survivor. If you can survive what you have been through, well, this should be a breeze." *Breeze. That's it! It's a breeze.*

Suddenly my spirit was lifted. Barbara didn't understand fully what she had said. A breeze. I remembered the sailboats, the wind. When the wind is the strongest, I can feel His presence the most. With His wind at my back, I can move forward. It is all in how I choose to look at it. *This is just another breeze! I can make it work for me.*

I needed the energy from the wind. My office looked like a hurricane had flown in. It was a mess. Barbara and I spent a couple of hours rearranging and redecorating. It was the same office, but the witness would be different. Yes, I was the same person, but my perspective had changed.

Tuesday came too soon. I entered McDonald's in a navy suit, tailored starched cotton shirt, and navy pumps. I had my brief-case, white journal, devotional book, and pens. I stood in line with the white-collar bunch of my North Dallas community. Sarah did not recognize me at first.

"Marsha, is that you?"

"Yes, friend. We need to talk."

I drank my coffee and desperately wrote to the Father while I waited for Sarah.

> Dear Father:
>   I need a word from You today. How will I tell Sarah that my life will be different now? Will she reject me when she finds out I am really another white-collar worker who has been playing "ragpicker"? Let my love convince her that I will never change. Let Your power make that true. I commit my life, my spirit, and my very soul.
>   As I reenter my old world, may the reflections of your Son be so evident. May Your name forever be glorified. May my life be a signature of Your love. It is in Your name that I sincerely write, for I am sincerely Yours.
>   Love,
>   Marsha

Sarah not only understood; she was thrilled. "Imagine, a 'white collar' loving me. That makes me special."

Sarah and I agreed to continue our coffee-cup ministry. We both had to adjust. Sarah took breaks earlier. I got up earlier. I soon learned that by getting up at 4:30 AM, I could walk, dress for work, and arrive at "my sanctuary" by opening time. I couldn't spend the entire morning, but I could spend nearly two hours studying and loving my friends. At 8:20 AM, I refilled my coffee and love and left for the condo to meet Barbara.

I was right. Nothing was the same. It was better. To the friends at my office, I soon became known as the "new Marsh"! To those at the "sanctuary under the arches," I was somebody special—their friend. I did not have to give up the good to have the best. I already had the best. I had been transformed. And only a transformed life had room for both!

Reflections on Love

The golden glow from within is a reflection of love. Just as the sun caused a golden effect on my skin, the Son caused a glow within.

Love is the total absence of fear. Love joins me to others. It is like a metal alloy or a strongly woven garment—love extended, expanded, included, and joined.

How did spending time in my secret hiding place change how I felt about love?

Love is choosing not to judge anyone's life but to see everyone in the light of forgiveness—even Jeff. It is choosing how I will face my fears. Love is the immediate peace that will always come the instant I choose not to judge.

Love allows everyone and every situation the opportunity to be my teacher. So, everything that ever happens to me is an opportunity to learn or teach love.

Only when I love myself can I love others. Love makes no comparison with the past. Love lives in the present.

I am never in need of love. I already have it totally inside. For He is love. I recognize love only as I give it away. The more I borrow from my storehouse of love within, the more it grows.

Love is a real emotion. Its voice can always be heard. I must always listen in love. So, rather than seeking solutions, I need only to seek to love. Love does not preclude action. Love makes my actions peaceful.

As I learn to love, I learn who I really am. Living is love. This is freedom. As I choose to love, I am choosing to live one moment at a time.

Unconditional love excludes no one. Unconditional love is giving without expectations. Unconditional love is total acceptance of ourselves and others without qualification, reservation, or the desire to change others.

In love, we seek only to accept and experience God's love. In love, we strive to express our gratitude to the good and Perfect Giver of love by giving His love away.

How do we live a transformed life of love?

1. We give up the need to be perfect by human standards. Instead, we seek only to let the Father be perfectly at home within.
2. We forgive and let go of the past. We view our pain as a possibility for growth.
3. We let go of prejudice. Every one and every situation in life can become our teachers. We decide.
4. We let go of pain to make room for growth. It can cut us or serve us. Again, we decide.
5. We seek solitude to breathe in His love and to recognize the love that is already within. We are made complete in Him.
6. We remember that fear is an opportunity to recognize that His light does burn brightest in the night.

7. We are patient. Positive change takes time.
8. We trust that love will never fail.
9. We seek humility. We are not afraid of feeling lack and limitation. Instead, we choose to let the voice of love transform these feelings into fullness and wholeness.
10. We accept all. Love can only influence those to whom we demonstrate acceptance.
11. We can make love our purpose for living.
12. We find a secret hiding place within our hearts to recognize and nurture His love.

(Based on notes from Gerald G. Jampolsky, MD)

Epilogue
A Time to Speak

Epilogue

June 29, 1987

Dear Father:

We did it! The book is finished. Sometimes I wonder if this is Your idea? I must admit that I have felt very exposed. I feel my private world is now an open book for the entire world to see. I wrote things in this manuscript that I had never before said to anyone but You. I feel almost naked. I even feel a little insecure, realizing that those who know me best will read this. Yet, Father, I am confident that if this is really from You, I will not be seen but You alone. This is my prayer.

There were moments in which I questioned if I were really following Your leadership in writing, especially on the day that I lost chapter 4 three times in the computer! But even that turned out well. I needed to think through that chapter more than once. I am continuing to learn from yesterday's experiences.

Yes, this book must be from You. Otherwise, I could not have managed the painful memories. It has been exhilarating. Each morning at 4:00 AM, the absolute certainty to write greeted me and my computer with words, wisdom, insights, and courage to climb out of bed. Maybe I know myself better since I have finally written it out. You did teach me earlier that I will know myself best when I can say what I mean. And, if no one ever reads this manuscript, I am confident that the discipline of having written is worth it all. I fell in love with You once again. I recognized Your magnificence anew. The timing was perfect for me.

Another affirmation was Mother and Barbara. I am still overwhelmed with their reaction when I told them of this project. Barbara said, "I have known for three years that one day you would write. Marsh, God wants to say so much through your life." And then Mother—well, You remember that she cried. You know so well that she saved every letter from ICU, as well as every piece of correspondence between us over the past three years? She, too, expressed that she knew it was just a manner of time until the book came out of me.

The timing is special. Even as I write, I am waiting once again. What seemed to be an ending may have only been a beginning. Even though it has been over four years, I continue to struggle physically at times. Will this always be the case? Maybe—maybe not. But in waiting, I have learned to lean and learn. I have gained a new appreciation for life, timing, relationships, and You. We have learned a great deal over these three years regarding the reason for my illness. Many discoveries have been made that link it to the preexisting conditions or even a virus, yet many questions remain unanswered.

Why is it, Father, that knowing is so much more comforting than not knowing? Isn't not knowing faith? If it is, my life will always be a walk in faith. It is faith now that makes the difference. I know that winter always follows summer and fall. Just because I have won some battles doesn't mean I will never have to fight again. Last winter's win (wind) cannot carry me through this season's storm. Something is different this time. The Son is shining. I know that there is nowhere I can go where You will not be. Oh, Your timing is so special!

These months of writing have prepared me to face the daily storms of life with security. They have helped me remember that the harder the wind blows, the farther I can move forward. Yes, Father, I know that yesterday's win (wind) cannot carry me through this season's storm. But I do know that the same Power that carried me through yesterday's winter will greet me with warmth. Seasons of my soul may come and go, but some things will never change.

So, for whatever reason I wrote this, I know I shall once again not only survive but be transformed in the winter.

Love,

MARSHA